THE PRACTITIONER AS TEACHER

THE PRACTITIONER AS TEACHER

Edited by

Sue Hinchliff

Scutari Press · London

© Scutari Press 1992

A division of Scutari Projects, the publishing company of the Royal College of Nursing.

First published 1992
Reprinted 1994

British Library Cataloguing in Publication Data
Hinchliff, Susan M.
  Practitioner as Teacher
  I. Title
  371.1

  ISBN 1-871364-70-1

Typeset and printed at Alden Press Limited, Oxford and Northampton, Great Britain

List of Contributors

Editor: **Sue Hinchliff** BA RGN RNT
Director of Studies, Distance Learning Centre
South Bank Polytechnic
Course Director—Diploma in Professional Studies in Nursing

Pauline Anforth RHV DipN(Lond) RGN RCNT RNT BA(Nurse
Education)
Head of Project 2000 Implementation, Stockport, Tameside and Glossop
College of Nursing

Terry Chandler RMN RGN DipN(Lond) CertEd RNT
Director, Staff Development and Training, Stockport, Tameside and
Glossop College of Nursing

Hilary Hampson BEd(Hons) SRN SCM FETC RCNT RNT CertEd
ICCert
Development Officer, Quality, Assurance and Research, Stockport,
Tameside and Glossop District Health Authority

Sally Thomson MA(Ed) BEd(Hons) RGN RMN RCNT DipN(Lond)
DipN Ed(Lond)
Lecturer in Education Studies, Institute of Advanced Nursing
Education, Royal College of Nursing

James Vaughan RMN RGN FET(Cert) RCNT CertEd RNT BEd(Hons)
MPhil
Vice-Principal, Post-Registration, Stockport, Tameside and Glossop
College of Nursing

Contents List

Preface

The impetus for this book came from two points. The first arose from my current post as Course Director for the Diploma in Professional Studies in Nursing by distance learning. On this course the students study a pair of units entitled *The Reflective Practitioner*, during which they are presented with material on a variety of themes relating to reflective practice, such as coping with stress, improving communication skills, becoming more competent at reflecting on what they do as they do it as well as after it's done, becoming professionally more assertive, improving decision-making abilities and so on.

While we were planning the curriculum for these units it became clear that we should be offering the students a learning package on how to develop their skills in teaching their colleagues, patients, clients and relatives and furthermore, how to reflect on these developing competencies in order to build on them. And so the idea for a distance learning package on *The Practitioner as Teacher* was born.

Since all the chapters have been written by different authors, you may perceive some differences in style and approach. I have made no attempt to edit these variations out. The whole tone of the book is that of a teacher talking you through the topics being discussed, and as all teachers have different teaching styles, I felt that you should be exposed here to such variety. You will notice that the book is written in the first person, that is, in a personal tone, rather than in the more formal style that you are used to in academic texts.

I was concerned that the book adopt an interactive format, where readers are urged to reflect on what they are reading, question their practice, examine the theory behind interventions, try out new approaches, etc. In fact, I saw the emerging package not so much as a book but more as a workbook, a resource to be actively *used* rather than just *read* and not just used once, but referred to many times throughout practice.

It is for this reason that you will notice that we have included quite a lot of 'white space', that is, space within the text for you to add your own notes as you read. I am aware that some of you will see it as verging on the sacrilegious to write on a book, but I am encouraging you to do just that here! Use it to jot down your responses to the activities that we provide. It will be useful to be able to refer back to them later. This book should end up as a very personal document, which records your progress in becoming a competent teacher.

Please don't try to save time by skipping the activities. Each one has been designed to make a point that will be learned more effectively by completing the activity. You will note that each one is followed by a comment, but that there are no right or wrong answers, just as there is no one right way to teach a topic, but lots of individual approaches.

With regard to the structure of the book, since all readers will be familiar with the nursing process, I decided to use that systematic approach here. The chapters are of equal importance, even though they are not of equal length. The book opens with a chapter on the nature of teaching and learning, to set the scene. It continues with four chapters which focus on:

- assessing learning needs
- planning for teaching
- the process of teaching
- evaluating teaching and learning

It concludes with a chapter which draws the threads of the preceding material together, in applying the contents to the practice setting.

Suggestions for further reading are included at the end of each chapter, annotated to indicate their usefulness and what the reader might hope to get out of them. At the end of the text you will find a composite glossary of words with which some readers may be unfamiliar. To indicate that a word appears in the Glossary, it is printed in bold where it first appears in the text.

We wanted the book to be equally useful, whatever the clinical speciality of the reader, whether a midwife, a nurse caring for old people, or a community psychiatric nurse and to be relevant at any stage of practice. I hope it will be used during courses leading to registration, for I have long felt that we leave learners somewhat in the lurch when it comes to teaching. They may know *what* to teach but strategies for getting the message across effectively are often not imparted until towards the end of, or after training, by which time many opportunities may have been lost.

A note about terminology

We have tended to use the term **teacher–practitioner** throughout, to denote the person who is doing the teaching. This term was chosen to indicate that the teacher is primarily a practitioner rather than a trained teacher. For the person who is being taught, we have most commonly used the word **student**, whether that person is, in fact, a student of nursing or midwifery, or is a patient, client or relative.

We have tried to avoid the use of gender-specific language, without resorting too frequently to cumbersome combinations of 'his/her', etc. Where the masculine or feminine pronoun has been used, this should not be taken to imply that a person of that gender is the usual occupant of the position referred to.

Whoever uses this book, in whatever circumstances, I hope that you will gain enjoyment and expertise from doing so. Above all, I hope that it will serve to open the door for you to some of the excitement, challenges and satisfaction that teaching has to offer. In both teaching and learning there's a lot of fun to be had, once you become confident enough to let yourself experience it. This book is designed to give you that confidence.

Sue Hinchliff

Chapter 1

The Nature of Teaching and Learning

Introduction

Regardless of whether you practise as a nurse, midwife or health visitor, situated in a GP practice, community or hospital setting, teaching is an important aspect of your role. Your student may be training for one of the registers, a patient or client, a relative, a colleague undergoing an orientation programme, a new doctor in the team or a member of the ancillary staff. Regardless of who the student is, they are entitled to the best possible standard of teaching that you can offer.

Teaching is a behaviour open to wide interpretation; it is something that can be developed and refined by improving your knowledge base, practising and reflecting on your practice. This chapter sets out to help you to develop a personal working definition of teaching, and considers the qualities of both effective and ineffective teaching as a basis for analysing ways to develop your teaching style.

Teaching cannot be considered in isolation from how people learn. We will link different teaching theories to models that will help to structure your teaching. A brief consideration of factors that affect learning will allow you to maximise every teaching opportunity that you have.

Finally, a framework for integrating all the ideas is suggested as a way of structuring the teaching programme in your practice setting.

Note that the words which appear in bold type throughout this chapter are explained in the glossary, which can be found at the end of chapter 1.

1.1. THE NATURE OF TEACHING

You may already feel comfortable and reasonably confident in your teaching role, or be at the other extreme, beginning to consider how you can develop this aspect of your work. Regardless of where you are in terms of insights into teaching, you may not have thought before about what teaching is. This may be a good point to start.

Activity 1.1.

Think either of yourself when teaching, or a colleague, and note down the behaviour that tells you that teaching is taking place.

You may come up with some conflicting ideas. Also note down any ideals or values that you believe are inherent in the word 'teaching'. Now compare your ideas with the following definitions.

Peters (1977, 151) provides a useful starting point for a definition of teaching. 'It includes a host of activities that have in common the structuring of a situation in such a way that something can be learned.'

The use of the word structured suggests a planned, rational approach, so that even if a situation demands that you teach in an impromptu way, you would stop for a couple of minutes, collect your thoughts, assess the resources available to you, think about what your student needs to know, and assess their readiness to learn before you begin.

But teaching is not as simple as that. Gage (1978) suggests that, like nursing, it is both an art and a science. The rationality of teaching theories could be viewed, for example, as the scientific approach, e.g. using a model of teaching that matches the style of learning, whilst the art may rest in the use of an analogy to illustrate an idea or the way in which the teacher relates to the students, sensing when someone is confused in a seemingly intuitive way, or in the use of a particularly imaginative introduction to a topic.

Lawton (1987) portrays the educator as one 'who enriches the life of a child across a wide range of worthwhile experiences'. We need to substitute 'child' for whoever our student is. It may be useful to consider what a worthwhile experience might be. In professional practice we have the opportunity to create experiences which can enable students to marry theoretical concepts to the practicalities of reality. A student may have a knowledge of sociology, psychology and physiology, and she may be able to write an essay discussing principles of rehabilitation for a patient who has lost a limb. Think, though, how much more real her perception of need might be if she accompanies an occupational therapist on a home visit with the patient before he is discharged; she becomes more aware, then, of the problem of how to get to a downstairs bathroom in the night, or of the psychological implications of needing two legs to pursue employment, e.g. a policeman. I doubt that you would disagree that this is a worthwhile experience.

A more difficult consideration may be the student nurse on a medical ward placement who asks for a teaching session on orthopaedics when you have no patients within this category on your ward. Is it worthwhile to grant her request? You know she is near finals; or may it be more worthwhile to use the opportunity to discuss a nursing problem which is currently common to several patients in your care, and which applies the theoretical knowledge gained from a study day? A difficult dilemma. Lawton then, may give food for thought.

The notion of what is worthwhile may be further explored by considering the influential work of Rogers (1983, 18) who states: 'the primary task of the teacher is to permit the student to learn to feed his or her own curiosity.'

There is a wealth of potential learning in each clinical area that your students can explore if you have the skills to facilitate this and if this is what your students want. Different students may be ready to be curious at differing stages in their course. Capturing the moment when a student knows what she needs to know is important. If, for instance, a student is experiencing referrals in her practice assessments, can you justify her desire to read about alternative methods of pain control when her drug administration is unsafe? This brings us back again to the debate of what is worthwhile and what you believe the nature of teaching to be.

For an inspiring and enjoyable read, do try Rogers (1983), who describes how a teacher can build on student-centred approaches to teaching with case study examples. This work is considered a classic, and is written in a style that makes it easy to dip into.

Now compare the ideas discussed so far with your own thoughts and the notes you made on what teaching is. You may have listed behaviours, such as questioning, that are inherent in the definitions we have discussed. These are, of course, just a few examples from the numerous differing definitions to be found.

You are probably beginning to realise that teaching is rooted in a value system. Your thinking may be in line with mine, or your ideas may be completely unrepresented in the discussion so far; neither of us is wrong. Teaching is a highly personal, and at times, emotional activity. What we all have in common is a marvellous grounding for teaching, from our experience, knowledge, beliefs, ideals and attitudes and from the rich resource of the practice setting in which we each work.

The primary aim of teaching, then, is that in a variety of ways, when it happens, it helps others to learn (Joyce and Weil, 1986).

1.2. CHARACTERISTICS OF AN EFFECTIVE TEACHER

Before reading on, think about a teacher that you would classify as good, or even brilliant. Jot down what it was about him or her that was so influential. How do your thoughts compare with the points below?

In general education, the qualities necessary for effective teaching have been widely researched. Good teaching is promoted by a sound knowledge base (Alulinas 1978, Fontana 1972, Henry et al 1981 and Schonell 1962). Ted Wragg (1984), in a down to earth mood, holds that the teacher should know her stuff; Sherman and Blackburn (1974) call for intellectual competence. It may also be important for practitioners to be aware of the things they do *not* know, particularly in caring settings where treatments and practices are changing so rapidly.

The good teacher develops a feeling for the students' emotional needs, social background and cognitive development (Fontana 1972). An interest in the welfare of pupils promotes learning (Wragg 1984). This is particularly pertinent to health care settings where 'pupils', regardless of who they are, will come from a wide variety of backgrounds, cultures and all age groups, so we have to be adaptable to meet such diverse needs. An insight into who your student is and how she is may help you get the teaching/learning climate right.

Henry et al (1981) found that the personal background of the teacher affected performance. Alulinas (1978) discovered the teacher's level of intelligence to be significant. It is not essential to know everything or be very clever, but it helps if you can assess whether the student is able to follow your line of thinking or if she is completely confused by the variety of interesting facts put before her.

The philosophical stand of the teacher is important (Henry et al 1981, Wragg 1974). Fontana (1972) calls for a unified philosophy of life. The teacher you have referred to may be someone who believes that the relationship with the student is equal, that learning is best achieved by doing something interesting and that students deserve respect.

Peters (1977) refers to the idiosyncracies of the successful teacher personality. The profile of characteristics highlighted in the literature are many. They include patience, consideration, emotional stability, maturity and sound judgement (Alulinas 1978). Wragg (1974) describes an unconventional, experimenting, flexible character; perhaps this is someone who is willing to break from the traditional methods of teaching. Fontana (1972) feels personal curiosity is important. This may be the teacher who works with the student to discover facts, experiences and relationships between events rather than telling the student what these are.

Significantly for health professionals, Wragg (1974) found that those teachers who offer minimal criticism and maximise pupil responses are favoured. This is difficult to transfer to one's own practice. Constructive criticism is a vital aspect of the teacher's role. If we do not help the student to identify areas where she has the potential to develop good as well as to correct negative behaviour, we cannot help her to maximise strengths and minimise weaknesses. Perhaps we ought to ensure, when giving feedback to students, that we balance the points on which to improve with the strengths. Additionally there are times when an unconditional 'that was excellent' without a qualifying 'but' ought to be used. Often if you ask a student if she is aware of the areas where she needs to improve she will tell you.

Before we point out the strengths and weaknesses of others, we may wish to demonstrate insight into our own potential and limitations. Fontana (1972) indicates that self-awareness predicts successful teaching, and may lead to a confident and assured manner (Sherman and Blackburn 1974) in your teaching style. Not surprisingly, a sense of humour is important together with a dynamic, pragmatic and approachable air (Schonell 1961).

Alulinas (1978) stipulates communication skills, verbal ability, interactive skills and calls for physical energy and drive!

Discipline, hopefully, is something that we will not have to worry about except in rare circumstances. However, in our practice we do need to be aware of the appropriate relationship boundaries.

Finally, researchers believe an enduring enthusiasm for teaching (Fontana 1972, Wragg 1974), an interest in the subject and the creation of an effective teaching environment indicate success (Wragg 1984, Sheffield 1974).

From the pupils' perspective, an effective teacher is one who gains credibility from competence, character and intention, is honest and fair, qualified by experience to know what she is talking about, and a person who is concerned about the students as well as self. Additionally, the teacher must be 'personalistic', remembering details of the students, as well as being sensitive to their mood and feelings (Burns 1982).

In nurse education, Howie (1988) describes how role models were chosen in the clinical setting because they were able to communicate effectively and appeared enthusiastic about nursing. Wong (1978) identified nine categories of teacher behaviour considered helpful to student learning.

1. Shows a willingness to answer questions and offer explanations.

2. Treats students with interest and respect.

3. Uses encouragement and praise.

4. Informs students of their progress.

5. Uses humour.

6. Has a pleasant voice.

7. Is accessible to students.

8. Supervises effectively.

9. Expresses confidence both in self and student.

Marson (1982) collected 49 statements about the characteristics of trained nurses considered to be good at teaching. These covered five areas:

- professional qualities
- managerial abilities
- personality traits
- empathetic qualities
- teaching abilities.

The report is interesting reading.

A study of perceptions of best and worst clinical teachers in a Faculty of a Canadian university (Morgan and Knox, 1987), revealed that the best clinical teachers were perceived by Faculty and students as good role models, who enjoyed nursing and teaching and were skilled and confident in both activities. They were approachable, promoting 'mutual respect'. Students perceived the best teachers as enthusiastic, non-belittling and encouraging independence. The Faculty valued breadth of nursing knowledge, clear explanation and ability to increase students' interests as important features.

Burns (1982) advocates that effective teachers have positive self-concepts, believing that how teachers perceive themselves and students will determine the effectiveness of their teaching. He refers to Combs (1965), who lists eight features of the effective teacher. He or she:

1. will have an internal (from within self, i.e. ideas and values) rather than external (e.g. pressure from peers) frame of reference, seeking to understand how things seem to others as a guide for behaviour.

2. is more concerned with people and their reactions than with things and events.

3. is more concerned with how things seem to people rather than facts.

4. seeks to understand the causes of people's behaviour in terms of current thinking, feeling and understanding, rather than in terms of forces exerted upon them now or previously.

5. trusts others and believes people have the capacity to solve their own problems.

6. sees others as friendly and enhancing, rather than hostile or threatening.

7. sees others as worthwhile.

8. sees people and their behaviour as developing from within, rather than from the result of external events, e.g. nurses work to give care rather than for financial rewards.

Burns (1982) concludes that how teachers perceive themselves and others will affect their ability to teach.

Are the behaviours that you listed as qualities of a good teacher reflected in any of these research findings? You may find that your definition of teaching in the first activity has crept into your thoughts as you have read this section.

1.3. THE INEFFECTIVE TEACHER

As we have seen, the criteria for an effective teacher are wide and varied. It may be useful to consider behaviour which does not facilitate learning in an attempt to narrow the field.

Student teachers who failed a course of teacher training in general education had difficulties with classroom management (which we might substitute for clinical area), were unable to relate well to students, displaying poor teaching methods, and had a lack of commitment to the profession (Rickman and Hollowell 1981).

Alulinas (1978) describes plodding, self-conscious, nervous, easily-tired student teachers who were insensitive to learner needs and had a weak impact upon them. Alternatively, the ineffective teacher may be 'big mouthed', outspoken and disruptive, frequently displaying behaviour which goes against the organisational norm.

Similarly in the nursing literature, ineffective teaching results when there is a lack of interest from qualified staff, who may distance themselves physically and psychologically from the students (Marson 1982). The trained staff may pose a threat when teaching (Wong 1978), so that students are unable to relax sufficiently to enable the kind of dialogue necessary to allow learning. Trained staff may demonstrate a lack of enjoyment of nursing (Morgan and Knox 1987), and be unwilling or unable to answer questions and insensitive to students' needs (Marson 1982).

Wong (1978) indicates that staff who act in a superior manner, belittling students or supervising them too closely, are not successful teachers. Personality clashes may also affect learning (Marson 1982), although this is not something that can be necessarily avoided. Morgan and Knox (1987) describe poor teachers as being deficient in communication skills.

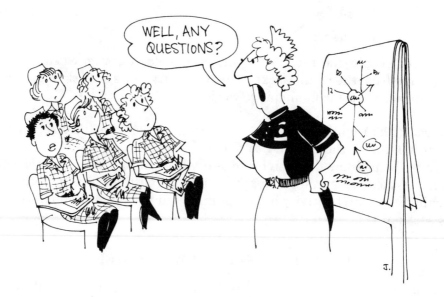

Whilst in general education lack of criticism of students is seen as a feature of poor teaching, in professional nursing literature unsuccessful teachers tend only to emphasise the students' mistakes and weaknesses, correcting in the presence of others (Wong 1978), or may be unable to identify objectively students' strengths and weaknesses.

Burns (1982) links unsuccessful teaching to poor self-concept, stating that teachers who feel personally and professionally inadequate and who dislike teaching, may be easily distracted and indifferent to pupil performance. Furthermore, they tend to act in a hostile manner, tending to control the teaching situation.

As can be seen from Table 1.1, many of the features of successful teaching are linked to positive relationship skills; similarly, ineffective teacher behaviour is often linked to poor interpersonal skills and an inability to respect and value the student. Table 1.1 contrasts 14 features of the ineffective teacher, with 14 identified features of the effective teacher.

Table 1.1. 14 traits of ineffective teachers contrasted with 14 effective traits of effective teachers.

Ineffective teacher traits	Effective teacher traits
poor classroom management	good role model
poor relationship skills	good interactive skills
poor communicator	good communicator
lack of commitment	enthusiastic
plodding	energetic
self-conscious	self-aware
insensitive	sensitive
outspoken	emotionally stable
disruptive	considerate
disinterested	curious
distanced	accessible
threatening	fair
superior	appropriate
belittling	encourages

1.4. WHERE ARE YOU IN THE EFFECTIVE TEACHER–INEFFECTIVE TEACHER CONTINUUM?

Having read this brief review of the literature, you might be feeling that the good teacher has a wealth of characteristics that are beyond your grasp! Remember though that the good teacher is not perfect, and the good teacher has bad days. There is plenty of room for all types of teacher, and indeed, if you compare your ideas of good teaching with that of a colleague, you may both come up with very different types of ideal teacher and such variety is welcome.

Activity 1.4a.

At this point, take some time to consider how many positive teaching characteristics you possess. Some things are difficult to change, such as intelligence and personality, but you should be able to develop and maximise your strengths when teaching, practising consciously the things you do well.

If you are concerned about your teaching skills, try to read the appropriate chapters in one of the books on communication style that are suggested under Further Reading. It may be helpful to focus on empathy, effective listening and questioning, exploring the use of such skills in your clinical work.

You may also find it helpful to develop a few ground rules to avoid falling into the ineffective teaching trap. For example:

1. when giving a student feedback on her performance, always begin with the things that he/she has done well;

2. avoid pointing out errors or reprimanding in front of a patient or colleague;

3. call errors 'points to consider', try to focus on two or three major points, setting goals for improvement;

4. offer students your time: 'we could have fifteen minutes this afternoon looking at this';

5. always say when you do not know, and suggest ways of finding out;

6. observe the student sensitively, and see if the response to 'how are you?' matches what you see, if not explore further.

Finally, it is important that you develop a perceptive and objective self-concept. It is all too easy to evaluate a teaching session that you have just done in a negative way, focusing on the less good aspects at the expense of celebrating the things you did well. If you genuinely value your own strengths you will value what you see in others.

Although some people seem to be born teachers, the complexity of behaviours that constitute teaching can be learned and developed.

Activity 1.4b.

Write down one thing that you are good at as a teacher and which you would like to build upon.

You may be surprised at the strengths you possess. We will be referring to this later in the chapter, but meanwhile try to be aware of this aspect of your behaviour as you go about your work.

1.5. FACTORS AFFECTING LEARNING

Imagine the frustration of executing a perfect piece of cognitive teaching, to find that the student is so anxious about getting her work done that she has been unable to attend to your session.

Child (1986a) suggests that the teacher should consider cognitive entry characteristics, in order to make an assessment of the student's or client's intellectual abilities. This is particularly important if someone is over-whelmed by the anxieties of a new ward, or by the implications of a recently divulged diagnosis. It is also important to establish previous experience, determining whether or not the subject has been taught in the college, or by a colleague, and exactly what the student knows about it. Similarly, it is important to find out just how much the patient/client knows, so that you can build on this past experience to extend understanding and create new insights. Marson (1982) found that trainees often reported teaching experiences coming too soon to be assimilated, as they lacked the necessary background knowledge and experience. Benner (1984) found that 'capturing' a patient's readiness to learn forms a key feature of effective teaching. Similarly, past experiences of teaching sessions may influence the student's perceptions of your role. Students may have had negative experiences which may interfere with your session, until they realise you have a different approach.

Communication skills (Child 1986a) are crucial in the teaching process. If your student has sensory impairment or limited vision or speech, you will have to be very sensitive to his or her feedback to ensure that she/he is following and understanding.

Affective (i.e. emotional) characteristics will also impinge upon the teaching and learning process. The student's self-concept will influence her approach to her learning. If she has recently been referred in an assessment or is repeatedly experiencing failure, she may believe she is incapable of the work and block her learning. Prompt feedback from you on her successes, pinpointing areas where she should concentrate in order to improve performance, will help the student develop a more realistic self-concept.

Motivation influences learning and this is strongly affected by the student's degree of interest. You can increase motivation in practice settings by helping the student gain a sense of achievement as he/she integrates theory and practice. Motivation will be reduced, regardless of interest, if your teaching prevents the student from completing planned client care on time.

Anxiety may affect learning. Some of the best performances are under-taken in anxiety-provoking situations; however, if the degree of anxiety becomes intolerable, the student will be unable to learn. A student caring for an extremely sick client may be able to improve care once you have provided a rationale for the various bits of equipment she is expected to use and she can see them in the context of the patient/client's care.

Personality may affect the process of learning. Marson (1982) found that personality clashes were a significant deterrent to learning. Similarly, someone who has an extraverted personality may enjoy sessions with distractions and digressions whereas a more introverted person may be annoyed by these.

Embarrassment and discomfort may interfere with learning. The student who is taught or reprimanded in front of a client may fear that the client realises how little she knows; admitting you do not know can occasion discomfort and embarrassment. Similarly, a patient may not wish to be taught in front of visitors.

Remember, too, that tiredness, pain, hunger or feeling unwell will all affect a person's ability to learn and develop. Atkinson et al (1990) provide an account of Piaget's stages of concept formation. A person who is anxious, unwell or tired may move back (regress) to a stage of concept formation characteristic of a younger age group. To teach effectively, you may have to pitch your session in more concrete terms than you would have thought necessary in order for clients or relatives to understand.

The key to minimising the factors affecting learning is to treat the learner as an adult (unless they patently are not!), use negotiation,

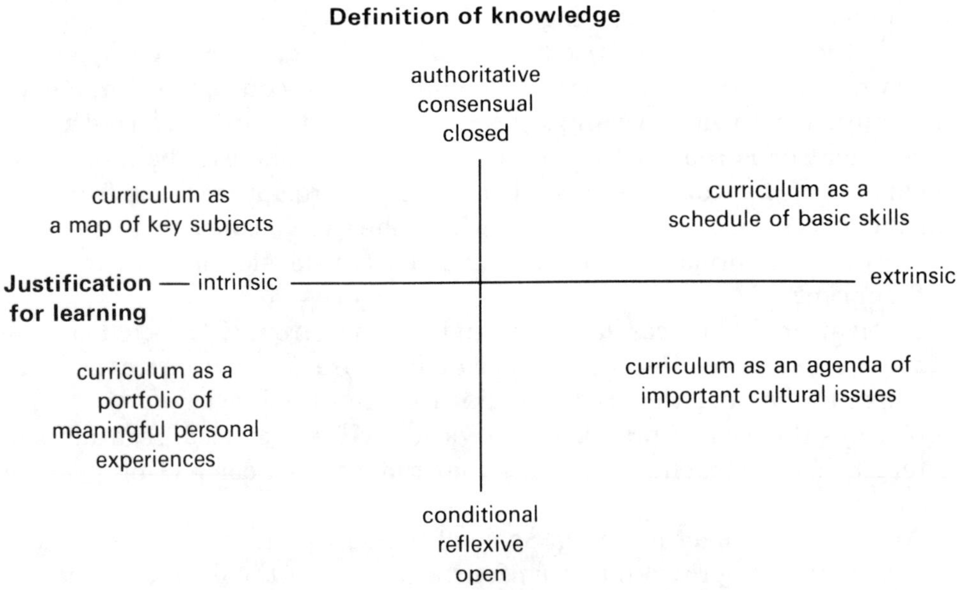

Definition of knowledge

authoritative
consensual
closed

curriculum as   curriculum as a
a map of key subjects   schedule of basic skills

Justification — intrinsic ————————————————————————— extrinsic
for learning

curriculum as a   curriculum as an agenda of
portfolio of   important cultural issues
meaningful personal
experiences

conditional
reflexive
open

Figure 1.1. The fourfold curriculum (from Beattie 1987).

establish past cognitive and emotional experiences and draw and build upon these, making clear links relevant to experience.

1.6. A FRAMEWORK FOR THE ANALYSIS OF TEACHING

Beattie's (1987) 'Fourfold Curriculum' model provides a useful framework for the analysis of four different learning theories and four ways of structuring teaching. The model is shown in Fig. 1.1. It is based on two axes. The vertical axis reflects definitions of knowledge ranging from authoritative, consensual and closed (for example, facts which have been proven by research such as the physiological events in the cardiac cycle), to knowledge which is conditional, reflexive and open (for example, the experience of conducting a first delivery which has the potential to be different for every midwife). The horizontal axis places learning somewhere between intrinsic and extrinsic. The two axes form four boxes which lend themselves to four different approaches to **curriculum** planning, and in our case, four ways of approaching learning and teaching, which we can now examine.

1.7. THE CURRICULUM AS A MAP OF KEY SUBJECTS

The curriculum as a map of key subjects would include a blend of biological, psychological, nursing, midwifery, medical and sociological sciences. In the practice setting, threads from these disciplines are drawn together to make the theory–practice link. These disciplines form the knowledge base that informs practice. For example, without an understanding of the physiology of the cardiovascular system, it would be difficult to give a patient, who was being discharged on digitalis, effective and safe advice on taking the drug; similarly a new mother who wishes to breast-feed needs to be given information relating to her nutritional and fluid requirements.

In order to teach these subjects effectively, it is necessary to understand both the perceptual processes involved and **cognitive learning** theory. Cognitive learning theory emphasises active participation of the individual and recognition of information in order to acquire complex information.

Perception

The **cognitive school of psychology** (practitioners of which believe that the mental processing of thoughts affects learning) suggest that learning can be stored in memory, retrieved and used in a new way when needed. Whatever the teacher intends the student to learn, the latter will make her own approximations according to the way she perceives stimuli, and what she has stored in memory from past experience and learning that is associated with what is being taught.

Followers of the **Gestalt school of psychology** talk about **perception** in relation to pattern perception. They describe four important features which make up the law of Pragnanz, the perceptual process. The principles of this process have great relevance to the way teachers structure their sessions.

The first principle is *similarity*. We need to form similar elements into a pattern of shape, size and colour. In teaching we can use this principle by beginning with what the student knows. For example, a relative asks for an explanation of her brother's pleurisy and the symptoms he is experiencing. You ascertain that she has little knowledge of body function. You might begin by likening the pleura to a skirt with a petticoat underneath, the two layers gliding upon each other smoothly as the lungs move with breathing. The petticoat develops static electricity and the smooth movement of the layers is disturbed. You could move on to explain that the pleurae are sticking together not because of static electricity but as a result of inflammation and this prevents their free movement and this is causing the pain. Analogies, then, have a useful place in enhancing perceptual processes.

Proximity, the second principle, is when similar objects appear close together and enhance accurate perception. In teaching we could compare how like one thing is to another looking for similar and contrasting properties. Suppose you are teaching a student nurse or midwife the principles of wound management, to enable her to care safely for patients. You could begin by carrying out an aseptic technique on a patient or client with a small sutured wound; next you perform a dressing for a patient with a corrugated drain in situ, then together you check the vacuum on a closed drainage system. At the end of the morning, you sit down together and look at the principles of care involved for the three patients/clients, comparing and contrasting the caring actions and emphasising the common principles of care.

Continuity occurs when similar parts of a figure, which appear in straight or curved lines, seem to stand out so that the pattern is evident. Continuity can be achieved when teaching by following a theme with your student, by moving sequentially through a topic in a logical manner. As an example, a wife is getting ready for her husband's return home from hospital following a fractured spine which has left him quadraplegic. Last week a staff nurse taught her how to prevent constipation. Today, to achieve continuity, you are going to focus on ways of managing bowel evacuation so your teaching is still linked to elimination needs, which you will ensure she understands, before moving on to discuss hygiene needs, or their sexual relationship.

The fourth principle of the law of Pragnanz is *closure*, which focuses on the fact that closed or partially closed figures are easier to perceive (the principle used in joining up dots in children's comics). So, by closing a teaching session using a summary, or any other technique which allows integration of the material contained in the session, you will help the student complete the perceptual pattern, tying all the threads together.

It is evident that by reflecting on how a learner organises information and by using the principles of the law of Pragnanz, we can make teaching more effective. If you wish to read more about perception, the chapter on this in Atkinson et al (1990) is enjoyable (see Further Reading at the end of this chapter).

Learning By Problem-solving

Myles (1989) describes how cognitive learning requires us to process the information received actively and transform it into new knowledge and categories. Its prerequisites are, therefore, the mental processes that perceive sensory inputs, the ability to encode it, store it in memory and retrieve it for later use.

Gestalt psychologists use the theory of insightful learning which builds on the theory of perception. They describe insight as the sudden solution of a problem by perceiving the relationships essential to the solution. This may occasionally occur dramatically, and people often seek the experience of insight by completing crosswords, for example.

Kohler, a Gestalt psychologist, used chimpanzees to demonstrate the nature of problem-solving. Sultan, the chimp, is in a cage; through the bars and out of reach is a piece of fruit, inside the cage is a short stick, and outside the cage, again out of reach, is a longer one. He tries to reach the fruit with the shorter of the two sticks, and frustrated, he tears at the netting. Next there is a long pause while he gazes about him, scrutinising the area. Very purposefully now, the chimp uses the short stick to secure the larger stick which he uses to reach the fruit. From the moment he began the activity his movements became one consecutive whole (Child 1986a).

Sultan was also able to transfer this learning and with the stick was able to reach fruit hanging from the ceiling of his cage.

Trial and error learning may be evident at the beginning of problem-solving, but once the task is seen as a whole it can be restructured in ways which affect solutions (Atkinson et al 1990).

The structure of the problem dictates the nature of problem-solving in Gestalt psychology. If a student is placed in a situation in which she/he has no knowledge, learning has to be by trial and error, and the patient on the receiving end of this may experience problems in their care of a more or less serious nature. If a student is presented with a problem for which it is possible to have a mental image, she may find a solution more easily.

Gestalt psychologists suggest that the efficiency of learning is dictated by the perceptual context in which learning takes place. They suggest that we learn by insight, using problem-solving.

Teaching By Problem-solving

Myles (1989) refers to Fox (1975), who cites seven steps to problem-solving and links it to Kohler's experiment. Do read the chapter in Myles (see Further Reading), before considering the applied example below, in which you are helping a student to plan care.

1. *Problem*   A client who has been severely depressed following a still-birth but who is beginning to recover asks to visit her baby's grave.

2. *Data collection*   Consider the situation and alternatives, her physical well-being, the motivation for the trip, her mood, the journey, etc.

3. *Hypothesis formulation*   A visit to her baby's grave would be therapeutic.

4. *Select plan for hypothesis testing*   What caring interventions may be necessary? Do you need medical consent? What if something goes wrong? Planning the journey (the what, where, when and how's).

5. *Test the hypothesis, implement the plan*

6. *Interpret results*   It went well, the client returned looking tired yet relieved.

7. *Evaluate the hypothesis*   She has asked to go next time with a relative (so it is evident the trip was therapeutic).

The student will have cared for a patient outside the security of the ward environment and will have insight into the detailed planning necessary for arranging such an activity.

The approach may look simplistic and if it is, cognitive activity may have been minimal. Ornstein (1990) has some useful ideas for developing problem-solving skills; he refers to Cybert's (1980) ten steps.

1. Keep the basic problem in mind and avoid distractions. In the example given, you may need to forget problems of staffing, pressures of ward routine, etc.

2. Avoid early commitment to a hypothesis.

3. Simplify the problem by using phrases, symbols or formulae.

4. Change an approach as soon as you can see that it is not working.

5. Ask questions and attempt to answer them.

6. Be willing to question assumptions.

7. Work backwards, if necessary, to work out solutions.

8. Keep in mind practical solutions that may later be combined.

9. Use metaphors and analogies.

10. Talk about the problem.

This approach moves problem-solving away from the realm of a superficial guessing game and provides a structured framework within which it can take place.

Before you can begin problem-solving, the learner needs relevant information in order to assess the situation. In the example described, this may be a knowledge of the effects of depression and grieving, an awareness of drug interactions, the client's history, etc., which will form the prerequisite information. The more able you are to help the learner set the problem in context, using concrete examples, the better able he or she will be to solve the problem. Having solved the problem, you may then help the learner to apply concepts (this worked for Mrs Green, what about Mr Brown?) so that she/he is able to generalise and adapt his or her professional practice.

Activity 1.7a.

Now try out this approach for yourself. In the group of clients that you and a learner are caring for, identify a client problem that is fairly common, albeit for a variety of reasons, e.g. difficulties with breathing, or painful wound healing or poor self-image. Select one patient/client for whom this problem is a priority.

1. State the problem:
    What information does the student need in order to work out solutions? Are there any exceptional or irregular circumstances to be taken into account?

continued on next page

continued

2. Use questions to draw on the student's knowledge base, and be ready to develop insight by offering explanations (**exposition**). Note below the key questions you might use.

3. Help student to collect all the relevant information she needs in order to state the problem (care-plans, drug charts, text books, etc.).

4. Brainstorm (without evaluating) as many possible solutions that you can think of with the student, writing them down.

5. In the light of the student's knowledge base: evaluate each idea; challenge, question and seek a rationale; ask for limits and constraints for the range of alternatives; and select the most feasible solution.

6. Plan jointly how to implement this.

7. Implement the plan. If it has not materialised as envisaged, return to stage three of this activity.

8. Evaluate the process together.

9. Ask the student to examine the appropriateness of the chosen intervention with other clients who have the same problem, to establish if the solution is open to generalisation.

Clearly, undertaking an exercise of this kind requires that you are able to work with the student for a span of duty in order to complete the suggested process.

Problem-solving is an easy exercise if it takes place at a superficial level; to achieve depth poses a greater challenge. You may need to use the technique yourself several times to get it right and to become familiar and comfortable with it.

Teaching by Using an Advanced Organiser

Ausubel, an educational psychologist, developed the notion of an advanced organiser to complement his theory that learning occurs through the interaction of new material with information already stored in memory (Myles 1987).

In order for learning to occur in a meaningful way, three factors have to be considered. Firstly, the student must have an appropriate learning 'set', that is a readiness to learn in a certain way. Secondly, the new material must have logical meaning, so that it can be related to the student's own cognitive structures in order to provide the foundations on which to build new material. Finally, the student's own cognitive structures (memory) must contain specifically relevant ideas so that new information can be integrated with it. Consideration of these three factors will mean that the teacher begins at the right level (Quinn 1988).

In this way, new ideas are not just added to the pile of old learning, but rather they become integrated with existing knowledge, skills or attitudes to form a new cognitive structure with greater meaning (Quinn 1988).

Ausubel's model is appropriate for teaching in the practice setting since it builds upon the involvement between student and teacher, it makes use of examples, and it uses deductive reasoning (knowledge gained by working things out). Finally, the model is sequential, beginning with an advanced organiser which links existing knowledge to new by forming conceptual bridges (Myles 1987).

Ausubel believes there is a parallel between the organisation of subject matter by the teacher and the way people organise knowledge in their minds, that is, their information processing system.

The model has three phases of activity: firstly, the presentation of an advanced organiser, followed by the presentation of the learning task, and finally the strengthening of the cognitive organisation (Joyce and Weil 1986).

The advanced organiser is an introductory statement of a high degree of depth that is broad enough to encompass all the information that will follow in the session (Myles 1987). Its purpose is to give students the information they need to understand the session, that is, it will help to 'create set'. The organiser will also bring to mind information the student already has that she/he may have thought irrelevant to the session. In this way the bridge is built between existing information and new material.

The organiser can be presented in several forms: expository, comparative (Joyce and Weil 1986) and diagrammatic (Myles 1987).

Take the example of a practice nurse setting up a slimming club for clients; the aim of her first meeting is to generate motivation to lose weight by explaining the effects that obesity has upon an individual. The

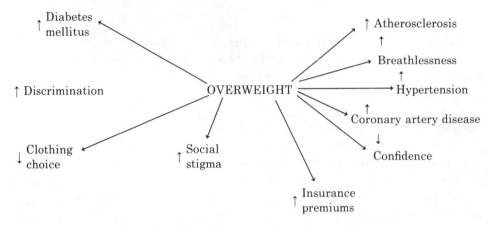

Figure 1.2. Example of an advanced organiser.

advanced organiser could be as shown in Figure 1.2. The subject matter may be organised with the use of a film, leaflets and group work.

The organiser is at a higher level of abstraction and inclusiveness than the learning itself, in that it explains, integrates and interrelates the material in the learning task with previously learned material (Joyce and Weil 1986, 76) so it provides pegs on which to hang the material that follows. The teacher, then, must help to explore the organiser as well as the subsequent learning. For instance, in the slimming group, the teacher will have to explain why the different diseases result from being over-weight. She may ask members what happens to their breathing if they run or climb stairs. Clients may disclose the medical problems they experience.

The learning task may involve explanations of energy intake and output, and the introduction of a diet plan that is restricted in calories.

To end the session and strengthen the cognitive organisation, she may emphasise the importance of weight-loss by revising the hazards of obesity, stressing that it is not too late to prevent further damage. She would ask students to summarise the key principles of the diet, repeating definitions and asking for differences between aspects of the regime.

Activity 1.7b.

Think of one topic or theme that is repeatedly taught in your clinical area. Make an advanced organiser for this, and outline how the session would evolve. You may find this quite hard to do. Practice will help you to develop this method.

This section has looked at the curriculum as a map of key subjects, examining how students learn and suggesting teaching models that will enable such learning to take place. It is crucial in this domain to build on the student's existing knowledge base.

Teaching strategies that are appropriate for use within the four models include exposition, use of question and answer, guided study with feedback, crosswords and quizzes, handouts (both written and diagrammatic), use of case studies, buzz groups, **brainstorming** and problem-solving.

Regardless of your practice setting, you should be able to build up a resource bank of visual aids to support your teaching, including textbooks, research papers and journal articles, diagrams, models, items of disposable equipment, in addition to mental models such as analogies. Finally, the value of the patient/client and of your own experience, in teaching, cannot be underestimated.

1.8. THE CURRICULUM AS A SCHEDULE OF BASIC SKILLS

This aspect of the curriculum is described by Beattie (1987) as those areas of practical competence which are:

> 'deemed to be essential for responsible and effective performance of professional tasks'. (Beattie 1987, 20)

In every clinical area there are skills which are either specific to that area or general to many placements. A complex matrix can be devised which illustrates the skills a student needs to master at each step of training, against the skills which are specific to the clinical context. In a surgical unit, a first ward student may be expected to meet a patient's hygiene and safety needs, in relation to preparation for theatre. A third year student may be expected to give total patient care, using the four stages of the nursing process and the framework of a nursing model with all the **psychomotor skills** that are subsumed within this.

In terms of patient/client teaching there may be skills which either a carer or the client has to be able to conduct, in order to be discharged into the community, e.g. a person with diabetes needs to be able to measure the glucose concentration of their blood, give insulin injections correctly, etc. A client with learning difficulties will have to master daily living activities, such as dressing, making drinks, etc.; a carer may need to manage emotional outbursts and unpredictable behaviour patterns. A new mother needs to feel confident in caring for her baby on a day-to-day level, managing baths and feeds. A client who is confused needs to be able to administer his own medication safely.

Learning From Behavioural Theories

These theories focus on the deliberate shaping of behaviour towards a desired goal. The **behavioural** school of psychology believes that the role played by the environment is crucial to learning. If the environment is structured correctly, learning will occur regardless of the volition of the teacher, as connections are made between **stimulus** and **response**, and response and **reinforcement**.

Myles (1989) identifies three 'key tenets' that form the basis of behavioural psychology:

- contiguity
- classical conditioning
- operant conditioning

Contiguity refers to the situation where, if two events occur together repeatedly, they will later become associated, so that when only one event is present the other will be remembered (i.e. the stimulus evokes a response). Myles (1989) stresses the significance of this in nursing when teaching and practising psychomotor skills: so that the correct sequence is always followed, the teacher should not encourage the repetition of inappropriate responses when someone is demonstrating a skill, as this destroys contiguity. Contiguity can be achieved by teaching skills in a systematic way.

Classical conditioning, made famous by Pavlov in the 1920s, focuses upon achieving certain reflexive responses by using stimuli. His famous experiment in which dogs were conditioned to salivate at the sound of a bell is an example of this. Myles (1989) suggests that this theory has little place in teaching, although original accounts of this work make interesting reading.

Operant conditioning, however, is a behavioural process that brings about purposeful actions. In this process, the animal (learner) is active and behaviour brings about important consequences.

Skinner is famous for his work in this field. In his experiments, a hungry rat is placed in a 'Skinner' box, which contains a bar with a food box beneath it. As the rat explores his new environment he occasionally presses the bar and everytime he does this, to his pleasure, a food pellet is delivered. This reward dramatically increases the incidence of bar pressing. If the food reward is not given the operant response (bar pressing) undergoes extinction. However, if a pattern of partial reinforcement is used, extinction of operant behaviour is usually much slower. There are important principles here for teaching. Firstly, if random behaviour is rewarded consistently, the incidence of that behaviour will increase; secondly, partial reinforcement delays extinction; thirdly, if behaviour is

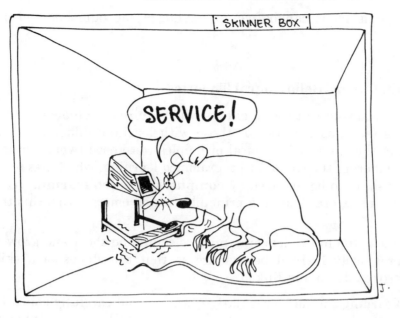

not rewarded (ignored) it is extinguished, a useful guideline for managing unwanted behaviour.

These principles can be applied to the child who has tantrums. If the parents occasionally reinforce this by giving in to whatever the child demands, they will receive more persistent outbursts than the parent who invariably gives way; whilst those who consistently hold out and refuse the demands enjoy the absence of such behaviour.

Operant conditioning plays an important part in the learning of new processes. Many driving instructors are expert in this approach. Often behaviour is shaped by positively reinforcing the subject as the behaviour gets nearer and nearer the desired response, such as reversing efficiently, or changing gear smoothly using phrases such as 'much better', 'nearly there'.

It is important to consider the set of rewards that you would wish to give. Some of you may have experience of caring for clients using behavioural regimes, such as **token economy**. Usually, in teaching, social reinforcers are used; these include nods, smiles, praise, eye contact, writing students' responses down and the verbal reinforcers of 'well done', etc.

The concept of punishment (although its place in clinical teaching practice is of little value) is an interesting issue; teachers punish using put-downs, sarcasm and by keeping students at a distance. Punishment decreases the probability of a response but it fails to give the learner an alternative choice of behaviour. The effects on the learner of the use of punishment can be worry, dislike of the punisher and deviant behaviour.

Teaching Using Behavioural Theories

Many of you who work with clients who require a high degree of skilled teaching (such as children or those with learning difficulties), will be expert in this field. Behavioural principles were used twenty or so years ago to underpin the trend for programmed learning, which has now gone out of fashion to be replaced by **computer assisted learning (CAL)**.

There are several teaching principles which emerge from this theory:

1. Each step in the learning process should be short and grow out of previously learned behaviours so that the stages of a skill are broken down and linked.

2. Learning should be regularly rewarded and carefully controlled by continuous or intermittent reinforcement (Child 1986). When teaching, you may move through a continuum from continuous to intermittent reinforcement. Social reinforcers, used in a variable ratio, are very positively received, and rapid feedback on a student's work will promote learning. Something as simple as 'you cared well for Mrs Jones this morning, she looks comfortable' has enormous potential as a reinforcer. Reinforcement can be used in this way to 'shape' behaviour. Shaping is an important concept. A shy student who has been allocated to your unit and receives positive reinforcement as she adopts the **group norms** is likely to settle quickly into her role. The principle of extinction may be useful if a student or client is displaying undesirable behaviour; ignoring the event serves to make it non-profitable, especially if acceptable behaviour is rewarded.

3. The reward should follow immediately after the desired response appears (Child 1986). Although this has been briefly mentioned above, in true behaviourism a delayed reward is meaningless as the reinforcement will not be linked to the operant behaviour.

Teaching Using Simulations

Some thirty or so years ago simulation had a high profile in professional education, with a large practical classroom in the school of nursing or midwifery which could be turned into an operating theatre or delivery room in minutes. Some of the more mature readers of this chapter may have been deemed fit to practice as the result of an examination conducted as a simulation.

Nowadays, simulations can be very sophisticated, relying on computer technology which can represent anything from the flight deck of an aircraft, to wind surfing. Similarly, situations may be enacted using board games (e.g. Monopoly simulates 'real-estate speculation', Joyce and Weil 1986). Conducting a simulation requires forethought, so that you have time to devise a game, or collect together the equipment, including any software that you might need.

The simulation model rests upon the principles of cybernetics: essentially a feedback system, which generates movement towards a desired goal, monitors errors and redirects behaviour.

A simulation has the advantage of making the learning task less complex than when it occurs in the real world. For instance, once the position of a proposed stoma has been decided, nurses can begin pre-operatively to teach a patient how to use appliances and manipulate equipment, establishing the best positions and practising without the hazards of a wound, drain site, rods, intravenous infusion and all the post-operative discomforts.

Similarly, students may 'fumble' with equipment on a resuscitation trolley, before they have to use it for real.

In a simulation, the student learns from direct self-generated feedback on crashing the plane or stalling the engine. In the simulations described in this chapter the student may need teaching help with feedback, as awareness and perception are not enhanced in a simulation (Joyce and Weil 1986). It is the principles of behaviourism which direct the student and not cognitive learning.

Within a simulation exercise the role of the teacher is very important. Because the student is so involved in practising the skill of the simulation he or she may not be aware of what he or she is learning and experiencing. The teacher, then, needs to bring the concepts and principles underpinning the simulation to the forefront of the student's mind and to elicit his or her reactions. Thus, when teaching the patient stoma management you may wish the patient to experience running around, lying or sitting with a full bag, with it pulling away from the skin. You will stress that in the real world, the consistency of the stool will be different but the weight will be the same. You may then explore feelings, anxieties, the cosmetic effect on appearance, etc. In midwifery you may demonstrate a bath using a doll, so that the procedure is learned in the absence of a wet wriggling baby.

In psychiatry, a carer may wish to **role play** a strategy that she intends to use with a client, i.e. she may wish to confront a woman that she believes has alcohol hidden on the ward. The simulation will allow her to check out and modify her tactics.

Similarly, if the simulation revolves around a game, the rules of the game need to be spelled out and on hand for checking.

If a team approach is used in a simulation, the teacher may need to act as a referee; additionally, activities such as coaching, offering advice, supporting or suggesting the way forward would all be appropriate within this model.

Finally, once the simulation is completed the teacher needs to create an awareness of the difficulties that may arise when using this exercise in a real situation (Joyce and Weil 1986). The student will learn from the direct result of the simulation and additionally and importantly, as a result of teaching interventions.

A simulation has four phases which guide lesson planning (Joyce and Weil 1986):

1. *Orientation*   Outline the topic and concepts to be incorporated into the activity and present an overview of the simulation.

2. *Participant Training*   Practise the skill.

3. *Simulation*   Then give feedback, evaluate, clarify any misconceptions.

4. *Debriefing*   Summarise events and perceptions, examine difficulties and insights, analyse the processes involved, compare simulation to real life, relate to clinical experiences or to the clients' expected progress.

Joyce and Weil (1986) suggest that the use of a simulation has the potential to create a sense of effectiveness, enabling people to face consequences, encourage an increase in knowledge, empathy, critical thinking, decision-making and finally concepts and skills.

Activity 1.8.

Below we have given you space to plan a simulation to use in your own work environment. For example, baby bathing, helping a client to cook a meal, scrubbing up and assisting a surgeon, assembling and using resuscitation equipment, rehearsing electro-convulsive therapy, helping a client to express breast milk.

continued on next page

continued

1. What activity do you intend to simulate? Note your intention in
    doing this, and any equipment, visual aids and resources that
    you will need. Remember that you need to cite here details of the
    environment that will be suitable for conducting the simulation.

2. Note key points for the orientation phase.

3. Outline the details of the participant training (**a skills analysis**)
    by breaking down the procedure into small steps.

4. Conduct the simulation, note key points for next stage.

5. Debrief: what was learned from the exercise?

6. Evaluate. Does the session need modifying?

Once you have completed the six stages, you have a workable plan
which can be used over and over again, perhaps with some minor
modifications as the situation differs.

Teaching Using Social Learning Theory

Social learning theory can be considered under the behavioural approach,
although to a certain extent it overlaps into the domain of cognitive
psychology.

Vicarious learning is also a feature of social learning theory and is
defined as: 'learning by watching the behaviour of others and observing
what consequences it produces for them' (Atkinson et al 1990, 425).

Learning by modelling views behaviour as a two-way interaction between
an individual and his environment. Complex patterns of behaviour can be
acquired in this way (Quinn 1988). Myles (1989) believes that emotional
responses can also be learned by modelling. At the beginning of the
chapter we asked you to identify the characteristics of an effective
teacher. If you described a positive role model, then he or she may be
responsible for an enormous amount of vicarious learning on your part.

Bandura (1977) describes four features of the model and observer:

- *Attentional processes*, i.e. the degree of interpersonal attraction (liking) between the model and observer, and how useful and distinctive the observed behaviour is.

- The frequency of contact with the model affects the adoption of the behaviour; similarly the observer's level of arousal and ability to process information will determine what is learned. Finally, learning will also be influenced by perceptual set (what the observer expects to see) and the amount of previous reinforcement.

- *The retention process* is the second characteristic of this model. Remembering the modelled behaviour is a crucial aspect of learning; **rehearsal** and repetition therefore are important elements.

- *The model has a motor reproduction phase*: i.e. the student enacts the observed behaviour and evaluates it in terms of accuracy.

- *Motivation affects learning*: the behaviour is likely to be learned if there is value in it and it has meaning for the learner.

Research indicates that the most influential models are seen by the learner as having status, power and prestige (Myles 1989). He also reminds us of nursing research that indicates how strongly nurses are influenced by colleagues, especially the ward sister (Fretwell 1982, Melia 1983). He makes two important recommendations that incorporate the principles of social learning. The first is the maintenance of high professional standards; the second is that teachers should only model behaviour that they would wish others to adopt.

A lot of the teaching that you do in this category may occur without your awareness. However, there are ways in which you can build up Bandura's principles, which the following example will demonstrate.

A student comes to you to report that during the morning, a patient (on an elderly care unit) has been weeping. This is quite unusual, for the gentleman is making a good recovery and is almost ready to go home. The student feels she is unable to meet his needs and asks for your help.

In terms of attentional processes, together you evaluate the situation and agree that the patient needs time to talk and express his distress. With the student you plan how this can be facilitated. Using question and answer technique, you help the student to revise the verbal and non-verbal strategies that indicate listening, and will help the patient to talk.

As you run through each strategy, you note a key word on a sheet of paper so that the student has access to it during the interaction. You encourage the student to observe you closely, noting how you use the strategies you have written down, and ask her to note the behaviours that you use which enhance the interaction and those which might inhibit it. You encourage her to write these down as well as any questions she may think of when at the bed-side. The student is then cued. As far as possible, you may rehearse by running through again the strategies you intend to use, then you carry out the planned care.

To activate retentional processes, you establish whether or not you found the cause of his distress. Then you ask the student to identify the strategies you used and evaluate their effectiveness, you underline each tactic on her handout as she mentions it and write an example of each under the heading. You may also look for behaviours that inhibited the interaction and discuss ways of minimising the effect of these.

To achieve motor reproduction, you ask the student to select two strategies from the list that she would like to develop. To achieve this you then plan an interaction with a different client, with the student initiating listening behaviours and you acting as observer or resource if needed. Together you then evaluate her performance, away from the bed-side.

Motivational processes can be activated by reinforcing the success of her interaction, explaining the difference the interaction has made to the perception of the patient and consequently his care. You may help her to identify a skill in listening which she has the potential to develop further.

The teaching and learning behaviours that exist within the category 'a Schedule of Basic Skills' are not the narrow field of activities that one might initially expect. Principles from this area lend themselves to teaching how to tie a shoelace, at one end of the spectrum, to assertion at the other. The strategies you might adopt include demonstration, supervised practice, simulation and role modelling.

1.9. THE CURRICULUM AS AN AGENDA OF IMPORTANT CULTURAL ISSUES

Viewing the curriculum as an agenda of important cultural issues helps us to focus on teaching about both long- and short-term dilemmas and controversies in practice, and may include practical and ethical debates. I am sure that in your working environment you can identify many issues that fit into this category. Similarly, clients or patients may need to be aware of issues surrounding choices they may make, e.g. in respect of treatment, such as consent to electroconvulsive therapy or induction of labour, organ donation, HIV testing, etc.

The teaching emphasis in this category is both social and democratic, in that students may work in groups to raise awareness of issues, which may have no easy solution. The teacher needs a high level of interpersonal skills to facilitate such sessions.

Teaching Using a Group Investigation Model

The model is based on democratic processes and group decisions (Joyce and Weil 1986). It stimulates enquiry in an atmosphere of reason and negotiation, as the students together try to work through problems and seek answers.

The teacher plays a facilitative role, focusing primarily on the group process, perhaps helping the students to formulate a plan, whilst acting as a source of knowledge and resources, and keeping the project within manageable boundaries.

The structure of the model is applied in the following activity:

Activity 1.9.

With your student group, select an issue which is pertinent to practice, such as the problem of gaining informed consent in emergency situations. Do think of an example from your own practice area, since it is important that this activity can be carried out with real benefit to your area and the staff involved.

1. Plan a short teaching session to explain the complexities of the situation, so that all aspects of the situation are outlined.

2. Explore the reactions to the situation and note these on a **flip chart**. (Keep a record in the space below.)

3. With the group, decide on ways in which the issue can be explored and organise how information will be collected, e.g. one student may go to the library to look for definitions, two students may issue short questionnaires to patients, one student may interview medical staff.

4. Allocate deadlines for this material to be collected.

5. At the next session, as the group members present material, ask questions, challenge the students to find their own answers.

continued on next page

continued

> **6.** Recycle the activity—does a new problem or activity emerge? (Joyce and Weil 1986). If, for instance, informed consent is pursued, it may be that you now need to consider the significance of how this is documented in your records.
>
>
> You have found the six steps demanding, in allowing students freedom to explore and debate.

The model may be one that is difficult to plan ahead for, since relevant situations tend to emerge without warning. However, this is not always the case.

Joyce and Weil (1986) suggest the model can teach cognitive knowledge as well as social processes. Additionally, such sessions provide a medium for fostering interpersonal relationships in the team as well as independence in learning and respect for the views of others.

The facilitator in such a model needs to have a knowledge of and access to varied resources. For example, you may know of key research reports, or journal articles, or be able to introduce the group to appropriate personnel who have access to information. Your negotiated role may be to invite an expert speaker who can offer a perspective on an issue the group are exploring, e.g. the chaplain may have relevant resources, or you may have a colleague with a philosophy degree who could help with an ethical dilemma.

The curriculum as an agenda of important cultural issues, relies on the teacher facilitating the exploration of uncertainties. The learning group may be students, clients in a support group, the multidisciplinary team, relatives or carers. Teaching methods may include projects, **syndicates**, case discussion or the use of **critical incidents**.

1.10.   THE CURRICULUM AS A PORTFOLIO OF MEANINGFUL PERSONAL EXPERIENCES

The distinction between personal and social learning is blurred, and you may well come to the conclusion that the concepts and principles embedded within each category influence and effect each other.

Beattie (1987) describes a 'portfolio of meaningful personal experiences' as being organised around the individual student's interests and needs. The intention is that the student will reflect upon practice and share the experience with others. Beattie goes on to describe how it can be used for professional, moral and personal encounters. Similarly, for the patient or client it may be an opportunity to explore the context of illness. The wife of a client diagnosed as schizophrenic, for example, may wish to explore the role of the Schizophrenia Society and take an active part in its work, so that she too is doing something that may promote awareness. She may need your skills to help her reflect on this role in a purposeful way. You might imagine a similar situation with the new parents of a baby with Down's syndrome.

Benner (1984) highlights the importance of reflection in her research, which uses the Dreyfus model of skill acquisition to demonstrate how students pass through five levels of 'proficiency' ranging from novice to expert. Benner's work clearly indicates the problem of the theory–practice gap, and is essential reading for anyone wishing to develop a teaching role in the practice setting.

The *novice* moves to a ward after a period in college, learning 'the rules' and principles of basic skills. These rules are inflexible and novice students are unable to contextualise them, that is, they are unable to make small adjustments to skills in order to apply them in practice.

The '*advanced beginner*' demonstrates a 'marginally acceptable performance'; Benner states that a mentor may have helped them cope with sufficient situations, issuing guidelines, to enable them to apply the rules.

The competent practitioner will have been in his or her role for two years or more; she/he is consciously aware of his/her actions, has a feeling of mastery but lacks the speed and flexibility of the proficient nurse. Benner suggests a mentor can enhance practice by using decision-making games and simulations that help the student to plan and co-ordinate complex care situations.

The proficient nurse has a deep understanding of the situation, in that she experiences it as similar to a past experience stored in memory and in this way a plan develops unconsciously.

The expert has an intuitive grasp of each situation and is able to select and analyse a problem without consideration of alternative aspects. An example is the sister who, seemingly intuitively, advises the night staff to watch a patient closely and predicts a sudden change in her condition, which materialises.

Schön (1987) would contend that personalising and reflecting upon experiences enables the student to transfer professional knowledge to 'real world practices', enabling the student to progress through Benner's five stages. Schön discusses at length the notion of professional artistry, calling it a form of intelligence, a kind of knowing, though different from professional knowledge. Artistry is demonstrated when competent practice is displayed in conflicting situations.

Schön (1987) calls this 'knowing-in-action'; he contends that 'reflection-in-action' will develop this professional artistry, so that a bridge is built between theory and practice. You may remember, at the beginning of this chapter, that teaching was defined as an art, hopefully within this context. Reflection, then, is something that you can facilitate in others and develop in yourself. Do read Bolt's (1991) work on *Becoming Reflective*.

Learning Through Personal Growth

This approach to learning is largely based on the influential work of Rogers (1983), who holds that education should 'facilitate the process of change in an individual so that she or he may function fully'. This is called a **humanistic** approach, in which the belief is that individuals are free to choose their own direction.

Rogers developed his ideas from his work in non-directive counselling. The approach is based on the assumption that learning is a development of self. Presuming that every individual has the potential for self-development, the facilitator attempts to reduce the differences in level of knowledge from what is known, towards the aspired level, which will help the client sort out his problems.

Rogers (1983) stresses the importance of the tutor–student relationship in which the student explores ideas about work and relationships with others and achieves personal integration, effectiveness and realistic self-appraisal (Joyce and Weil 1986). The approach depends upon students taking responsibility for their own learning.

Joyce and Weil (1986) summarise the key features of the humanistic approach:

1. Individuals have a natural drive to learn.

2. Learning can be maximised by using experience.

3. Self-evaluation encourages independence and creativity.

In order to bring about this type of teaching, the facilitator needs skills in building a lasting, non-threatening relationship, for example, in:

- listening and responding consistently
- helping the student to identify feelings and personal knowledge
- sharing of him/herself
- being sensitive to the student's needs

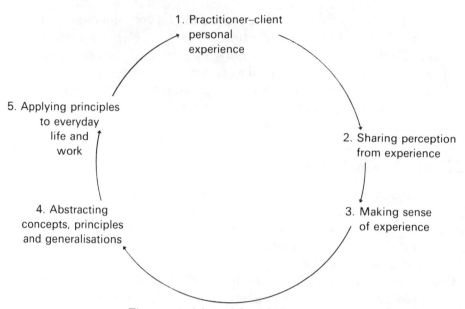

Figure 1.3. Adapted from Miles 1987.

- being aware of personal strengths and weaknesses and their effect upon others. This has links with Burns' concept of the effective teacher discussed earlier in the chapter.

Rogers (1983) tends to make the practice of such a style sound easy. As with other models, the development of this approach takes time and practice; the adoption of such a stand requires considerable reflection and personal development on the part of the teacher.

Teaching from a Student's Experience

Miles (1987) describes how the teacher can build upon the experiences of the student, using an experiential learning cycle. This can form a useful framework for maximising teaching in practice settings (see Figure 1.3).

An example of how the model might be used is when the 'Novice' (Benner, 1984) is caring for patients before and after gynaecological surgery. As a teacher, you are trying to help her apply the rules of pre- and post-operative care to a particular patient. Together you are planning care for a patient who is to have an abdominal hysterectomy. The patient is resting after premedication and you sit down with the student to explain the nature of the operation, using a labelled diagram. Together you escort the patient to theatre and remain with her during anaesthetic induction. The student remains in theatre, shadowing the charge-nurse to observe the operation and to monitor the care given in the initial stages of recovery.

Once the patient is back in bed and her present needs are met, you encourage the student to share her perceptions of her experience, perhaps with the other students on the ward. You may ask what she saw and felt. Initially the student may be overwhelmed by her initiation into the theatre environment: incisions, blood, smells, the beauty of the pelvic organs. She may, though, go on to describe how brutal retractors are; she may, with your prompting, recall the surgical procedure. As she talks, you write her perceptions down on a large sheet of paper using keywords.

In order to make sense of the experience, the student needs to understand what it all means, so that she can transfer this information to inform (that is, to illuminate) future post-operative nursing care. You revisit the key words on the **flip chart**, e.g. retractors, encouraging the student to work out the effect this has on the patient—she may identify bruising or stretching and you may then be able to demonstrate how this contributes to pain, discussing how the potential problems could be managed.

Abstracting concepts, generalisations and principles may be achieved by exploring the extent to which the other patients in your client group who have had a hysterectomy have experienced similarities and differences in their needs and planned nursing care.

The example given is concrete. The experience could with equal validity be the administration of the student's first injection, the first experience of induced labour, breaking bad news, handling an emotional outburst, etc. What is important is that the student agrees to the use of his or her experience for teaching purposes.

The potential of the model for client teaching is varied. Consider the person with newly diagnosed diabetes, who is to have a hypoglycaemic attack induced so that they and their family can recognise and manage the situation when it occurs.

Firstly, the patient and relatives should be prepared by explaining what to expect. The hypoglycaemic attack is induced and the patient is stabilised. You explore with both parties what was observed and what was felt. You are then in a position to make sense of the experience by linking what happened to altered physiology. From this you can deduce the features of a hypoglycaemic attack and how to manage it, deriving concepts and principles. Finally, you apply the principles to everyday life, coping with exercise, etc.

Teaching Through a Reflective Process

Boud et al (1985) describe a process which develops the learning experience using a reflective cycle (see Figure 1.4). The model has three phases, the experience, the reflective process and the outcomes.

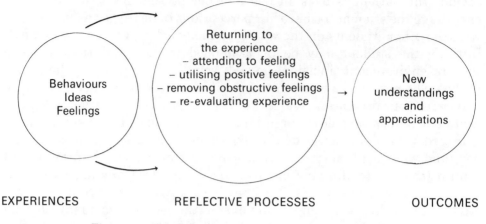

EXPERIENCES   REFLECTIVE PROCESSES   OUTCOMES

Figure 1.4. The reflective cycle (After Boud et al 1985).

The student, client or colleague identifies an experience which they wish to explore with you. They should be asked to reflect on the experience and to record the salient points, i.e. to replay the events. This account could be a verbal, written or visual exploration. The next step is to ask them to focus on the feelings associated with the experience in order to use positive emotions and to examine, remove or balance the effects of negative feelings. In re-evaluating the experience a re-examination of events in the light of reflection takes place to cement the learning that has occurred.

Let us take the following example to demonstrate the technique: A client, adapting to life in a self-propelled wheelchair, takes himself off to 'have a go' in the streets surrounding the hospital. On return to the ward over a much needed coffee, the two of you reflect on the process.

You begin by asking what happened. The client describes the positive side of his outing but states that he will only use the chair in his garden. It transpires that a well-meaning pedestrian, without invitation, has propelled the patient across a pedestrian crossing, disempowering him. Feelings such as anger, helplessness and embarrassment emerge. The client may be laughing or crying as his emotions are released. You may help him put his emotions in perspective by exploring how real they are. Who was staring? Was the pusher patronising or concerned? The client should be helped to see that he did achieve his objective and, if it is appropriate, helped to alter his perception. Importantly, you could help the client to identify strategies that would deter offers of unwanted help. In rehearsing some of these, he could judge their effects upon the would-be helper and in this way new outcomes to the situation may emerge. If the client does not work through his negative emotions, he will not adapt to the full extent of his potential.

Schön (1987) states that reflection helps others to make decisions under conditions of uncertainty. He suggests two ways of reflecting; firstly, by thinking back on an action, as described; secondly, by stopping before, or in mid-action to think, and generate a different outcome. In this way, professional and personal behaviour will become shaped and reshaped. If you think it necessary to stop a student in mid-action, do, but execute this away from the patient so that the student maintains her poise and the patient is unaware of any potential problem.

Activity 1.10.

1. At the beginning of this chapter you identified some of your strengths as teacher. Select a teaching session that you have undertaken in the past week. Write an account of the session. Pay close attention to detail, noting events that occurred and your reactions. Include recollections of judgements you made at the time, but try not to interpret your story just yet.

2. List the emotions and thoughts that you have about the session. Select the positive ideas and consider ways of maximising them in other teaching sessions. Now examine the negative feelings you may have. To change your perspective, imagine that in your place someone whom you think of as a good role model carries out your session in exactly the same way. She invites you to discuss her negative emotions. What interpretations would you put on them?

3. Consider ways of incorporating strategies into your lesson plan that will minimise these negative aspects in your next session.

Undoubtedly you will have found this exercise difficult to do at anything other than a superficial level unless you are comfortable with self-reflection. Reflection requires the development of habit. This may be acquired by writing a reflective journal, perhaps by focusing upon aspects of your role that you wish to develop, e.g. assertion or counselling skills.

Valuable personal experiences can be created in groups or in one-to-one

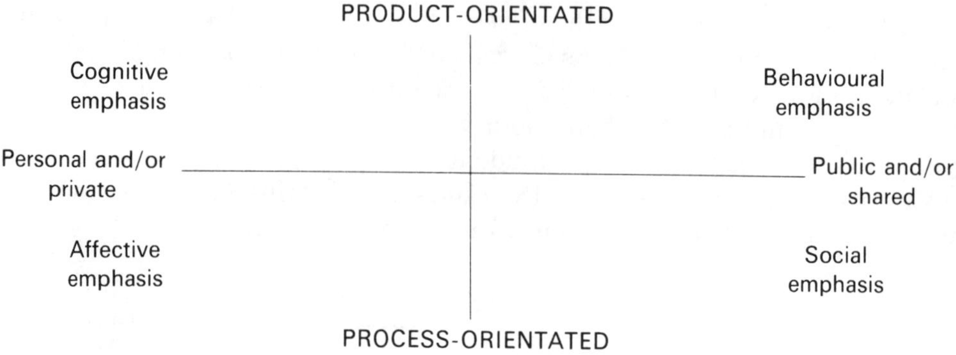

PRODUCT-ORIENTATED

Cognitive
emphasis

Behavioural
emphasis

Personal and/or
private

Public and/or
shared

Affective
emphasis

Social
emphasis

PROCESS-ORIENTATED

Figure 1.5. Alternative methods of teaching (Beattie 1986).

settings. You may discover a large overlap in this area with teaching that occurs socially, i.e. using the group investigation model.

Methods that help the student to learn and develop from reflective practice include reflection itself, the numerous activities that make up experiential learning, critical incident analysis, problem-solving, journal-writing, video feedback, **process-recordings** and discussion.

1.11.   TEACHING AND LEARNING USING THE FOURFOLD CURRICULUM

Figure 1.5 plots the four ways of approaching teaching that complement the four ways of viewing learning opportunities for any learner in your working environment.

If you have completed the activities you will now have lesson plans for each of the four approaches that you can use as a model for other sessions.

Activity 1.11.

Compare and contrast the four styles of lesson plan. What are the difficulties and strengths of each approach? How does the role of teacher and taught change with each type? How comfortable are you with these roles? You may discover that you are able to switch categories or that your work and style suit just one or two.

By now you will have realised that principles of behaviourism enter into your cognitive learning session as you smile, nod and value student contributions; cognitive strategies have crept into your skills teaching; personal and social learning strategies have fused together, personal learning enhancing cognitive teaching, so that the knowledge gained from each session interacts with, relates to and complements learning in the other three areas.

You may wish to reflect upon the methods you use most frequently, investing some time in studying the uses and abuses of all the different methods you could use, ranging from teacher-led to student-centred (Sheahan 1980).

How can you devise a teaching and learning programme in your area that meets the four requirements of the map of key subjects, a schedule of basic skills, a portfolio of meaningful personal experiences and an agenda of important cultural issues? You may already have identified learning objectives for students that work in your area. In most clinical areas, there are objectives for each student-year. The first year students may have to achieve objectives which are mainly skills-based; by the second year the objectives may have increased in breadth and depth to reflect the increasing experience and ability of the student; and third year students will be set increasingly complex outcomes to achieve. Whilst it may be appropriate for all students to achieve the same outcome, some students may wish to explore issues further. For instance, it may be a core objective that a first year student is able to assess the need for analgesia for a patient in pain. To achieve this the student needs to understand the effects of prescribed analgesics, and to perceive a patient's needs accurately whilst understanding the physiology and psychology associated with the experience of pain. If a learner achieves this objective, she has achieved a great deal. However, she may still be curious about pain relief, and may wish you to guide her studies further.

Similarly, you may need to consider the essential knowledge, skills, insights and personal learning that your client needs to adopt in order to make a healthy recovery. Remember, though, that some clients or carers may be motivated to learn more than you initially plan so you will, therefore have to adapt your teaching to meet their needs.

A common core curriculum (Lawton 1975) can work well, with all students working to achieve the same objectives at the same level. However, as discussed, some students may be satisfied with what they have gained in one area, but may wish for more depth in another.

Lawton (1975) offers a curriculum which lends itself beautifully to adoption in the practice setting (see Figure 1.6). On the matrix, the horizontal line labelled A–D represents the core objectives that you wish each student to achieve during her allocation to your area, or that a patient needs to achieve in order to adapt to his condition. These core topics may

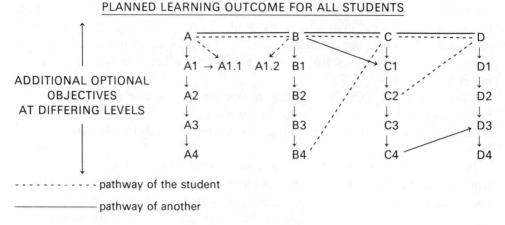

PLANNED LEARNING OUTCOME FOR ALL STUDENTS

ADDITIONAL OPTIONAL
OBJECTIVES
AT DIFFERING LEVELS

- - - - - - - - - - pathway of the student

———————— pathway of another

Figure 1.6. A curriculum matrix adapted from Lawton 1975.

be linked to the practice competencies, and embrace the knowledge, skills issues and personal developments which you hope all students will gain.

The vertical line represent additional objectives at a variety of levels and difficulties, which cater for the differing interests and abilities of the student group.

For instance, we have already discussed the core objective of assessing the need for analgesia for a post-operative client. A student may wish to explore the place of alternative therapies such as massage, or to consider how psychological interventions can help to alter perceptions of pain. To facilitate this you may need to devise some guided study, or a visit to a specialist nurse with a worksheet to complete.

Lawton suggests that for every core objective the teacher should work out additional themes at a variety of levels and difficulty, which cater for the differing interests and abilities of the student group. Some students will spend large periods of time and require skilled facilitation to achieve a core objective, whilst others climb down the ladder to gain more depth. The student who found difficulty in one area often seeks more information and discovery in another. In this way the richness of the clinical learning environment can be capitalised upon in a multitude of ways.

The drawback of such a model is the amount of detailed planning that is needed if the programme is to be successful. Each activity needs to be prepared so that the student is guided appropriately. Additionally, you may wish to structure activities so that as students move down the matrix, gaining breadth and depth, they move towards a student-centred approach. Strategies that you could prepare might include worksheets and diagrams, guided reading, visits with guidance to a medical museum, pathology laboratory, scanning department, etc.; you may set projects;

you may develop themes which focus on activities of living, or themes which underpin the particular framework for practice which is in use. Additionally, assessment, planning, implementation and evaluation may help determine levels especially when linked to Benner's (1984) stages of practitioner competence.

A group of you on the ward could get together to develop this idea. You should find that you can build on the learning opportunities that you have to offer.

CONCLUSION

This chapter has considered the nature of teaching, and the characteristics of effective and ineffective teachers. An overview of four approaches to teaching and learning has been presented, providing you with an opportunity to develop your ideas for teaching in each section. A way of structuring your teaching programme is suggested, followed by a brief consideration of factors that detract from learning.

The final task is to consider how you might develop your repertoire of teaching activities. Part of the answer lies in having a go, but understanding the knowledge-base that informs teaching, practising and developing your skills, reflecting on the practice of good role models will all raise your awareness of issues that impinge on your teaching role, and will result in your enhanced performance. You might apply the fourfold approach to yourself, by developing knowledge and skills, and by sharing teaching and learning with your peer group, reflecting with them and privately, and perhaps also with a mentor.

GLOSSARY

Behaviourism: the study of psychology by considering an individual's behaviour rather than the functioning of the brain and nervous system.

Brainstorm: an intensive situation in which spontaneous suggestions for solutions to problems are generated by a group, without evaluation. The group later evaluates the suggestions and decides on the best alternative(s).

Cognitive learning: considers that mental processes and representations are essential to learning so that we are not passive receptors of information but actively process incoming data, transforming it into categories and new forms.

Cognitive School of Psychology: an approach to psychology that stresses the role of mental processes in understanding behaviour.

Computer assisted learning: uses the principle of operant conditioning in which the student' correct response is rewarded with praise and encouragement via the computer software.

Critical incident: a snap-shot, a moment in time when an occurrence in the daily work of the carer will affect client care. Events may be large, small, positive or negative, e.g. a positive interaction between a client and carer.

Curriculum: the education programme of an institution which includes philosophy, teaching method and its implementation and effects.

Exposition: a period of teacher talk, in which knowledge is imparted or explanations are given.

Flip chart: a giant-sized note pad fixed on an easel, useful for summarising points during a session or for revision or the conclusion of teaching.

Gestalt School of Psychology: a psychological theory primarily concerned with perception, which emphasises pattern organisation.

Group norms: members of a group act and expect each other to act in a standard way, e.g. styles of dress, ways of interacting, etc.

Humanistic: emphasises the qualities that distinguish people from animals. This school considers a principal motivating force to be a tendency towards growth and self-actualisation.

Learning theory: theories that study how relatively permanent changes in behaviour occur as a result of practice.

Perception: how we come to know what is going on around us by interpreting what is happening in ourselves and surroundings using senses, expectations and experience.

Process recordings: a verbatim, serial account of an interaction between two individuals.

Psychomotor skills: learning skills and procedures, co-ordinating sensory stimuli to achieve purposeful movement.

Rehearsal: repetition of an item or aspect of behaviour can transfer it into long-term memory.

Reinforcement: reinforcing a response by the presentation of a stimulus that increases the strength of the conditioning, typically in operant conditioning it is in the form of a reward.

Role play: students act out specific social roles for the purpose of increasing insight.

Skills analysis: breaking down a skill into small steps, so that it reads like a recipe, each step forming a stimulus response association.

Stimulus-response: a view that all behaviour is in response to stimuli, e.g. our response to the sound of an alarm.

Syndicates: where students are divided into groups to work on the same or related problems with teacher contact as needed. The syndicate present a joint report for the whole group.

Token economy: a system of rewards structured into a programme in which tokens can be exchanged for personal effects, e.g. a client may be rewarded with tokens for dressing, making his bed and doing his laundry. These can be exchanged for items in the hospital shop. This system may be used for clients with learning difficulties or behavioural disorders.

REFERENCES

Alulinas W (1978) Some Case Studies of Unsuccessful Student Teachers: their implications for teacher education changes. *Teacher Educator*, **13**(3), 30–37.

Atkinson R, Atkinson C, Smith E, Ben D and Hildegarde E (1990) *Introduction to Psychology*, 10th edn. New York: Harcourt Brace Jovanovich.

Bandura A (1977) *Social Learning Theory*. New Jersey: Prentice Hall.

Beattie A (1986) *Curriculum Development for Health Studies: a foundation for nurse teachers. Blueprint for the future*. London: King's Fund Centre.

Beattie A (1987) Making a Curriculum Work, in Allan P, Jolley M (1987) *The Curriculum in Nursing Education*. London: Croom Helm.

Benner P (1984) *From Novice to Expert*. California: Addison Wesley.

Boud D, Keogh R and Walker D (1985) *Reflection: Turning Experience into Learning*. London: Kogan Page.

Burns R (1982) *Self Concept Development and Education*. London: Holt, Rinehart and Winston.

Child D (1986a) *Psychology and the Teacher*, 4th edn. London: Holt, Rinehart and Winston.

Child D (1986b) *Applications of Psychology for the Teacher*. London: Holt, Rinehart and Winston.

Combs A W (1965) *The Professional Education of Teachers*, Boston, Mass: Allyn and Bacon.

Cortis A (1979) Twelve Years on—a longitudinal study of teacher behaviour continued. *Education Review*, **31**(3), 20–218.

Cybert R M (1980) Problem-solving and education policy, in Turna D and Reif F. *Problem Solving and Education: Issues in Teaching and Research*, New Jersey: Erlbaum.

Fontana D (1972) What do we Mean by a Good Teacher? in Chanan D (Ed) *Research Forum on Teacher Education*, Windsor: National Foundation for Educational Research.

Fox D J (1975) *Fundamentals of Research in Nursing*, 4th edn. New York: Appleton Century Crofts.

Gage N L (1978) *The Scientific Basis of the Art of Teaching*, New York: Teachers College Press.

Henry J et al (1981) Evaluation of Teaching Skills. *South Pacific Journal of Teacher Education*, **9**(1), 61–65

Howie J (1988) The Effective Clinical Teacher: a role model. *The Australian Journal of Advanced Nursing*, **5**(2), 23–26.

Joyce B and Weil M (1986) *Models of Teaching*, 3rd edn. London: Prentice Hall.

Lawton D (1975) *Class Culture and the Curriculum*, London: Routledge and Kegan Paul.

Lawton D (1987) The Changing Role of the Teacher: consequences for teacher education and training. *Prospects*, **17**(1), 91–98.

Marson S N (1982) Ward Sister—teacher or facilitator? An investigation into the behavioural characteristics of effective ward teachers. *Journal of Advanced Nursing*, **7**, 347–357.

Melia K (1983) Students' Views of Nursing 4: doing nursing and being professional. *Nursing Times* June 1–7, **79**(22), 28–30.

Miles R (1987) Experiential Learning in the Curriculum, in Allan P and Jolley M, *The Curriculum in Nursing Education*, London: Croom Helm.

Morgan J and Knox J E (1987) Characteristics and 'Best' and 'Worst' Clinical Teachers as Perceived by University Nursing Faculty and Students. *Journal of Advanced Nursing*, **12**, 331–337.

Myles A (1987) Psychology and the Curriculum, in Allan P and Jolley M (1987) *The Curriculum in Nursing Education*, London: Croom Helm.

Myles A (1989) An Overview of Psychology as Applied to Nursing, in Hinchliff S M, Norman S and Schober J (Eds) *Nursing Practice and Health Care*. London: Edward Arnold.

Ornstein A C (1990) *Strategies for Effective Teaching*. New York: Harper and Row.

Peters R S (1977) *Education and the Education of Teachers*. London: Routledge and Kegan Paul.

Quinn F M (1988) *The Principle and Practice of Nurse Education*, 2nd edn. London: Croom Helm.

Rickman L W and Hollowell J (1981) Some Causes of Student Teacher Failure. *Improving College and University Teaching*, **29**(4), 176–178.

Rogers C (1983) *Freedom to Learn for the 80's*. Columbus, Ohio: Charles Merrill.
Schon D A (1987) *Educating the Reflective Practitioner*. San Francisco: Jossey Bass.
Schonell F J (1962) *University Teaching in Queensland* (Report of conference for demonstrators and lecturers). Brisbane: University of Queensland Press.
Sheahan J (1980) Some Aspects of the Teaching and Learning of Nursing. *Journal of Advanced Nursing*, **5**, 491–511.
Sheffield E F (Ed) (1974) *Teaching in the Universities: no one way*. Montreal: McGill University Press.
Sherman B and Blackburn R T (1974) *Eric Abstracts*, **9**(8), 88.
Wong S (1978) Nurse-Teachers' Behaviours in the Clinical Field: apparent effect on nursing students learning. *Journal of Advanced Nursing*, **3**, 369–372.
Wragg E C (1974) *Teaching Teaching*. London: David and Charles.
Wragg E C (Ed) (1984) *Classroom Teaching Skills*. London: Croom Helm.

FURTHER READING

Atkinson R, Atkinson R, Smith E, Ben D and Hildegard E (1990) *Introduction to Psychology*, 10th edn. New York: Harcourt Brace Jovanovich. Useful for revising or finding out about psychological principles.

Benner P (1984) *From Novice to Expert*, California: Addison Wesley. The research findings and use of the Dreyfus model of skill acquisition are essential reading and will help you better to understand your students. A valuable resource.

Bolt E (1991) *Becoming Reflective*, Distance Learning Centre, South Bank Polytechnic. An imaginative distance learning pack, which allows you to explore what it is to reflect in and on your practice.

Child D (1986) *Psychology and the Teacher*, 4th edn. An easy to read introduction to educational psychology. London: Holt Reinehart and Winston.

Fretwell J (1985) *Freedom to Change: The Creation of the Ward Learning Environment*. London: Royal College of Nursing. Essential reading about the role of the Ward Sister.

Hargie O (Ed) (1986) *A Handbook of Communication Skills*. London: Croom Helm. Providing an interesting and readable theoretical account of communication.

Heum C (1980) *Communication in Nursing Practice*, 2nd edn. Boston: Little Brown. This considers and applies communication skills to nursing.

Johnson O W (1990) *Reaching Out*, 4th edn. London: Prentice Hall. The book offers practical exercises which can help you develop your skills in communicating.

Marson S N (1982) Ward Sister—teacher or facilitator? An investigation into the behavioural characteristics of effective ward teachers, *Journal of Advanced Nursing*, **7**, 347–357.

Myles A (1989) An Overview of Psychology as Applied to Nursing, in Hinchliff S M et al (1989), *Nursing Practice and Health Care*, London: Edward Arnold. For a clear, succinct account of psychological principles applied to professional practice.

Rogers C (1983) *Freedom to Learn for the 80's*, London: Charles E McCall. Rogers describes one way of facilitating student-centred learning and the background philosophy. Worth reading.

Chapter 2
Assessing Learning Needs

Introduction

It does not matter whether you work as a nurse, midwife or health visitor in a community or hospital setting, assessment is an integral part of your role. Assessment may involve one of your patients/clients or, on the other hand, you may be assessing a student or a new member of staff. Whoever is being assessed, it is important that their level of skills and learning needs are clearly identified. This chapter addresses some of the issues surrounding the assessment process.

What is Assessment?

The term 'assessment' has a particular meaning for most people. The meaning placed upon it depends on your own personal experience, but unfortunately many people tend to associate assessment with determining levels of performance or achievement in a given situation. That is, the word has a strong connotation with 'testing'.

However, it is important to differentiate between two different types of assessment, that is:

- assessment that you undertake to establish what your students' learning needs or your patients'/clients' needs are. The purpose of this type of assessment is to establish a 'baseline' of future needs, and it is an essential prerequisite to planning teaching, or indeed, care. This type of assessment is often overlooked as there is a tendency to think of assessment as:

- a process by which a student's level of competence, achievement or performance is assessed.

The latter is associated with the assessment of performance during and after a student has been exposed to teaching, whereas the former type of assessment occurs *before* planning a learning experience. However, assessment should be an ongoing process throughout a teaching/learning experience, with students being encouraged to reflect on their progress both as and after they learn.

Activity 2.1.

Think of a situation where you were involved in assessing a student's or patient's/client's learning needs prior to teaching them. Note down all the points you can think of that you focused on. Alongside them make a note of the key skills that the teacher-practitioner should possess in order to identify these individual needs.

Amongst some of the points you may have noted down are:

- the behaviour of the individual being assessed, including their attitude to learning
- their apparent knowledge-base
- their likely facility with the material or skill being taught
- the context in which the learning is to take place
- your own behaviour and relationship towards that person
- your feelings towards the teaching situation, anxiety, uncertainty, etc.

Amongst the skills needed by the teacher-practitioner if s/he is to assess effectively are:

- self-awareness
- accurate observation
- ability to listen and interpret
- questioning skills
- sensitivity to the learner's behavioural cues
- ability to evaluate objectively.

All these factors will have played a part in your perception of the individual's learning needs.

Learning which begins with the experience and is then followed by reflection, discussion, analysis and evaluation of the experience, is called experiential learning (Wright 1970).

You seldom learn from experience unless you assess the experience and derive from it your own meanings, that is, make sense of it in terms of your own goals and expectations. This type of learning could be thought of as a meaningful type of discovery learning, as opposed to exposition, where the content of what is to be learned is presented to the learner, without the need to make corrections, make sense, interpret, reflect and evaluate.

Assessment of the Learner Within a Teaching Situation

Rowntree (1987) uses five dimensions in 'Assessing students: how shall we know them'. This text is included in the suggestions for Further Reading and is worth reading.

- Why assess
- What to assess
- How to assess
- How to interpret
- How to respond

If we examine briefly each of these given dimensions, it should be possible to get a comprehensive overview of assessment.

WHY ASSESS?

There are a number of reasons why assessment is used. The following are six reasons. There are many more you should be able to identify.

- To license nurses as competent practitioners—that is, we are required to assess learners at particular points in their education as a statutory requirement.

- To predict future behaviour—that is, assessment allows you to measure potential—what the learner might be capable of.

- To judge level of achievement—we need an accurate assessment of a learner's present abilities and knowledge-base in order to build on it in teaching.

- To monitor progress—assessment is necessary in order to judge how much learning and development has occurred.

- To motivate students—assessment focused constructively on a student's strengths, and on where improvements are needed, can be highly motivating.

- To measure 'teacher' effectiveness (Bligh 1972)—that is, the teacher needs some feedback on performance to see how effectively his/her planned teaching brought about learning.

WHAT TO ASSESS

- What the learner already knows; the range, level and depth of their knowledge and skill repertoire.

- The areas in which the student is deficient in the knowledge or skills needed for the job they have to do.

- The student's state of readiness to learn. Are they physically, psychologically and intellectually up to it? Do they possess the prerequisite manual dexterity to apply a complicated dressing? Do they possess the degree of self-awareness and sensitivity to counsel a patient/client with marital problems? Is a diabetic client able to work out the effects on his metabolism of drinking 2 pints of beer before lunch?

- To assess the learner's learning style. Do they learn best by chaining, linking one step of a skill, or one piece of knowledge onto the next —or do they learn best by seeing the whole picture first?

- To identify learning strengths and weaknesses. Do they feel more comfortable with the biological sciences or the behavioural sciences? Are they 'good with their hands'? Are they patient?

- The learner's level of motivation to learn and achieve. Is the learner well motivated in the clinical area or does s/he appear careless or disinterested?

- Is s/he confident or has s/he low self esteem? This may be evident from body language as well as from what the learner says.

These are all factors that should be assessed. How you go about assessing them will be addressed in the next section.

HOW TO ASSESS

When selecting the method by which you are going to assess your students, it is important to ensure that the chosen assessment method matches the content and style of teaching and learning experienced by your students, in order to avoid the use of inappropriate assessment methods.

One of the most commonly used techniques is the 'assessment interview'. There are numerous variables that you need to consider when using this approach. For example, is the environment appropriate and free from distractions, quiet, not too hot or cold and with comfortable seating?

Have you given some thought to the questions to ask and whether they should be open or closed questions? An example of an open question might be: 'What do you think might be the result if we do this?' or 'What do you know about . . . ?' The object is to obtain the views and opinions of the learner. Whereas, with a closed question you are looking for a precise answer, e.g. 'What is your name?' or 'How often should the insulin be given?'

Observation

You can learn a great deal about learners or patients/clients through direct observation of their behaviour provided that they are in their own familiar environment. Direct observation can provide reasonably accurate evidence of a learner's level of competence and performance. For example, you could assess a student's learning needs by observing him or her taking a patient's blood pressure. The observations should tell you how effective the student's psychomotor skills are, and you should be able to determine how confident she is and her general approach to the patient/client. You could also follow up your observations by spending some time questioning the student to establish their understanding of the skill and its underlying knowledge-base.

You may observe a student's performance in her clinical work 'unobtrusively'. That is, by watching her without her being aware of this. Through this process the student's normal work activities can be observed and assessed without interruption, and the student remains unaware of the assesssment. This tends to be an informal process and cannot be as objective as direct observation but it does represent how you see a student's behaviour at a particular point in time. While something can be learnt about a student's behaviour, using the latter approach, it should not become the only mode of assessment.

The presence of an observer tends to cause the subject to direct attention toward the self and to perceive herself as an object (Wicklund and Duval 1971). When this occurs, there is a tendency for the individual to compare her behaviour with standards of correctness. The result is that the learner will attempt to 'do her best' and make more of an effort to perform to a higher standard.

According to Bond (1982) individuals who perform in the presence of others are motivated by fear of embarrassment. They try to do their best to maintain face and an acceptable image. You might like to reflect on whether you agree with Bond and whether this applies generally within nurse or midwifery education and within your clinical area in particular. If this is so, try to think of ways in which such discomfort might be relieved.

When you are doing an assessment it is important that you try to remain as objective as possible. Total objectivity is difficult to achieve however. An assessor should be aware of his or her own prejudices, likes and dislikes, and try to avoid letting them interfere with the assessment process.

WHAT TO ASSESS

When deciding what to assess, Marshall (1960) suggests that a teacher should not record her opinions of a student using a prescribed checklist, prepared in advance and applicable to all students. Instead, the teacher should concentrate on what 'floats to the top' of her awareness as being pertinent to that particular student. The message from this is that if a teacher uses a rigid prescriptive framework, she is in danger of overlooking many elements that fall outside the criteria contained therein. A range of assessment tools, flexible enough to pick up the qualities you are looking for, is the most appropriate. Hopefully this way you will avoid what Holloway et al (1967) and Kelly (1958) observed, that students' personalities had an influence on teachers' assessment.

Activity 2.2.

Reflect honestly on a recent situation where you had to assess a student or a patient/client. Note down all the factors you can think of that you were conscious of when undertaking the assessment, which were not directly related to the assessment of the learner's needs. Next make a note of the steps you took, or criteria you used, to ensure that the person being assessed was not judged unfairly. For instance, how did you avoid letting your own values and feelings interfere with or cloud your perception of that person's needs?

Teachers sometimes make judgements about their learners which may or may not be complimentary, and it is crucial not to prejudge their needs and abilities on the basis of a chance remark, their apparent manners, their appearance or what someone else has said about them. When you are assessing the learning needs of your students, patients or clients, it is important to remember that your own level of knowledge and expertise is likely to be very different from that of the person you are assessing. You need to remember that the purpose of the assessment is to establish the student's learning needs before and during the teaching process.

Avoid comparing students with your own level of knowledge and skill. A clear understanding of the background and previous training, if any, that the person you are assessing has been exposed to, must be considered at all times. Reflecting on your own past experiences and how you may have felt if you were the person being assessed, can help you to empathise with the student. There are clearly many variables that can interfere with the assessment process; the more you as an assessor are aware of these and are able to control them, the more objective and accurate the assessment is likely to be.

When communicating to the learner your assessment of his or her needs, you should try to gauge, through the student's non-verbal communication, the response to your feedback. A face-to-face discussion also allows the student to seek clarification of any point which remains unclear. Always allow enough time for this, since it may take some students quite a while to come to terms with your assessment of need.

HOW TO INTERPRET

This is a very important part of the assessment process. Having noted and recorded all the data, the next stage is to make sense of what you have observed. The need for objectivity at this stage cannot be over-emphasised. A clear description of what you have actually observed or obtained by way of questioning is essential. Avoid making assumptions or inferences based on your own experience, colleagues' opinions or subjective impressions.

If you have been using criteria against which to measure the learner's needs, then there is a much greater chance that your interpretation will be more objective. For example, if you are teaching a patient how to change his colostomy appliance, then the criterion for day 1 of the teaching may be that he does no more than look at the stoma. By day 8, though, the criteria will be different and you might expect him to be able to change the appliance safely and hygienically. However, you need to ensure that if you are using some form of criteria-based tool for assessment, that it is both 'reliable' and 'valid'. Reliability refers to the consistency, stability and dependability of a measuring tool. Validity, on the other hand, means that the measuring tool should measure what it claims to measure.

The fact that you have recorded a particular incident or behaviour suggests that it is significant. You need to reflect on why you perceive it as being significant and if it is meaningful from the student's point of view. Only then can you use this assessment to plan your teaching effectively.

HOW TO RESPOND

The way in which you respond to what you have perceived and interpreted during the assessment, is very important. Giving feedback of good news on progress or performance is fairly straightforward, that is, pleasant both to impart and to receive. However, feedback that is more negative may be difficult for both the person giving the feedback as well as the recipient. As practitioner-teacher, you will, at some time during your professional career, have experienced being a recipient of negative feedback. Sometimes teachers adopt 'avoidance' tactics. Some readers may be familiar with what used to happen before it became a requirement that nursing students received feedback midway through their allocation. Many would pass through an allocation blissfully ignorant that their practitioner-teacher was dissatisfied with their progress. Then, having completed their allocation, they would have to return to sign their progress report, at which time they would be confronted with an unsatisfactory report. This was not only distressing for the student but was unprofessional on the part of the assessor.

Feedback, despite how painful it may be, is generally accepted if it is delivered in a constructive manner. The following are a few key points you need to keep in mind when giving feedback:

- Be sensitive to the recipient's needs, feelings and self-esteem.

- Start by focusing on the positive points—what were the student's strengths? What did s/he do well? Was her manner pleasant and professional?

- Try to be honest, fair and constructive—never be destructive—the whole point of feedback is to enable the learner to improve.

- Remain calm and try to be objective—do not respond in kind to aggression, anger, defensiveness.

- Allow the recipient of the feedback time to discuss and clarify any points they may wish to. This is crucially important and is often neglected in the teacher's rush to escape from a potentially uncomfortable situation.

Performance usually improves with feedback provided that the anxiety level is not allowed to increase *unduly*. However, to some students, knowledge of results presents a personal threat. Most individuals attempt to maintain an acceptable standard of performance and if they perceive this to be falling, they may become over-anxious. The increased level of anxiety may be exacerbated if the decline in performance occurs in the presence of a significant person. An example of this is a student who is carrying out a particular procedure or activity and something goes badly wrong while her supervisor or assessor is present.

SELF-ASSESSMENT

Self-assessment should be an integral part of all assessments. This should involve the person being assessed together with the person carrying out the assessment. If you recall, Wright (1970) referred to the importance of reflecting on, discussing and analysing an experience. Only by reflecting on experiences can you become aware of what you have really learnt, in order to put yourself in a position where you are able realistically to assess your development.

This reflective process leads to a gain in personal growth and self-confidence. Increased self-awareness should result in a clarification of learning needs. The process is highly individualised and the analysis of results are more meaningful and clearly understood by the individual learner.

Very often the teacher, as an assessor, is preoccupied with assessing the needs and skills of students, with the result that she fails to reflect on her own level of knowledge and skills. Self-awareness and a clear insight into how you adapt your own knowledge and skills to the needs of your students can only be gained through self-reflection on your own performance. Every experience should be a learning experience and practitioner-teachers should encourage and promote a critical, inquiring approach to their role by themselves and their professional colleagues and students. As a teacher with a critical, inquiry-orientated attitude towards your work, you have a responsibility to promote in your students a critical, inquiring attitude toward their learning.

Self-profiling has become a popular tool in the assessment of students (Coates and Chambers 1990). Through the process of self-profiling, students are asked to examine their own thoughts, acts, feelings, performance and responses daily throughout their training. The aim of self-profiling is to make the student into her own assessor. She is encouraged to be aware of her feelings, develop her strengths and critically evaluate her weaknesses which should then lead to realistic goal setting. This approach to self-assessment allows the student to develop greater insight of his or her strengths and areas where improvements are necessary, encouraging students to reflect on their progress and gains.

Activity 2.3.

Reflect for a moment on what you have read so far in this chapter.

Make some notes on how reflection and self-assessment could enhance your learning and further your knowledge and skills.

Having identified all the positive aspects that can be gained from this process, now think how you could put these into practice in your clinical area.

Much of the knowledge and skills we possess have been learnt from experience. According to Kolb (1984) people have a 'concrete experience', e.g. a student may experience a patient suddenly having a myocardial infarction in the clinical area where she was working. During and after the actual experience she 'observes and reflects' on what went on. This can be either a conscious or an unconscious process. As a result of her reflection and thinking, during and after the experience, she learns things which she can then formulate into ideas, knowledge and skills. For instance, having reflected on the part she played in the scenario described, the nurse may feel that she needs to increase her knowledge in certain areas, or may feel that another time she would plan to respond differently. The more often you repeat the experience, the deeper the learning should become. At the next stage, you automatically begin to start testing out your ideas.

Kolb's learning cycle (see Figure 2.1), using a self-reflective process, is attractive to students working in practice settings since it is simple, yet represents the experiential learning process realistically. You will notice the similarity of this figure to that presented in chapter 1 in section 1.2.

MOTIVATION

Motivation is central to learning and the advancement of knowledge and skills. There are a number of factors which play a part in our motivation. Maslow (1987) believes that people are motivated by physical, psychological and social factors. Our levels of motivation and its actual focus are determined by which factor is the most predominant at the time. As you will note as you study this book, the principles of reinforcement and

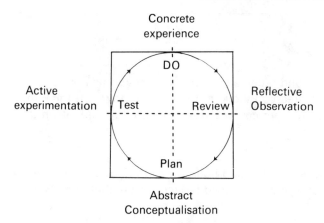

Figure 2.1. Experiential learning cycle (adapted from Kolb, Rubin and McIntyre 1971 in Boydell 1976).

reward are of crucial importance in learning. This, in turn, acts as a stimulus to students and provides the motivational drive to pursue new knowledge. The old cliché 'nothing breeds success like success' holds true. We all enjoy receiving positive feedback on our progress and performance. You have a key role to play in motivating students as a practitioner involved in the teaching and assessing of students in the clinical area. The following are some of the ways in which you can motivate students in the learning process:

• by providing psychological support and making learning 'comfortable',

• by enabling students to develop a reflective inquiring approach to the care they give,

• by providing feedback on their progress and giving positive 'strokes' as warranted,

• by being a suitable role model for students to strive to emulate,

• by providing challenge to the students, matched to ability, to stimulate and develop them.

These are just a few examples of how you could, in your key role, play an important part in motivating students in practice settings.

Maslow (1984) identified the fact that students' psychological needs (e.g. for stability, freedom from fear, reduction in anxiety) need to be met if motivation is not to wane. If students are feeling insecure or have high

---

Activity 2.4.

Having read and reflected on this section and its application to the practice area you work in, write down how you think the practitioner-teacher can act as a motivator for students in the practice setting.

Now think how you could build on all the good points you have identified and how you could reduce factors that demotivate students.

---

levels of anxiety, this in turn will affect their learning. Their concentration is likely to be affected, which will reduce their ability to take a critical inquiring attitude and reflective approach.

Only when students' self-esteem needs are satisfied will they feel self-confident, with a greater sense of self-worth and perceive themselves as being useful and effective practitioners. You, as a practitioner-teacher, can assess where a student is in respect of these needs. Your teaching and coaching can enable the students to develop insight and meet their individual needs.

Motivational drive to meet individual needs may be a conscious or unconscious process. Unconscious motivation is said to be associated with basic needs, e.g. hunger, thirst. Cultural differences play a part in determining the level of conscious motivational drive. This is important to bear in mind in the health care professions where the workforce is multicultural. Incentives and motivational factors that are the accepted norm in western society do not have the same effect on other cultures.

Vernon (1933) and Wolff (1943), cited in Maslow (1987), refer to two types of motivational behaviour:

- expressive behaviour; this type of behaviour does not set out to achieve anything, but is simply a reflection of personality, e.g. adults who behaves stupidly, not because they are trying to, or are motivated to do so, but as a result of a personality trait such as impatience.

- motivated behaviour where the behaviour is goal-orientated.

When assessing students' needs these are important factors to bear in mind if a true picture of learning needs is to be established. The relationship between needs and gratification is an aspect of motivation with which you need to be familiar. If you examine Maslow's hierarchy of needs, basic physiological needs dominate until satisfied and then the next most important area of need takes over until this is satisfied and so on. Maslow (1987) saw the layers of motivational need as:

- physiological
- safety
- affiliation—to be able to relate meaningfully to others
- self-esteem—to have a feeling of self-worth
- self-actualisation, i.e. intellectual challenge and self-fulfilment.

LEARNING ENVIRONMENT

This is a topic that has been much researched and written about (Ogier 1981, Fretwell 1982 and Orton 1981). The learning environment refers to wherever students are taught. However, as a practitioner-teacher your prime concern is with the practice setting. Teaching is about creating environments in which learning can take place and as a practitioner-teacher you are in a very powerful and influential position to do this. It is often said that a good classroom is one in which things are learned everyday which the teacher did not previously know.

We can all reflect on environments where we learnt a lot and felt self-satisfied and valued. There are many factors that are important in creating environments that are conducive to learning. A new or unfamiliar environment can be stressful enough by itself. If you then add other factors, for example:

- not feeling accepted as a member of the team
- being made to feel inadequate and foolish
- being given little guidance and support
- always being allocated the most unpleasant activities,

then the stress increases considerably and an environment that is inconducive to learning results. There are many reasons why a professional may behave in such a way as to create an unpleasant environment that acts as a barrier to learning. The individual practitioner-teacher may herself be stressed and that stress is then projected onto the student. The practitioner-teacher may have been exposed to this type of learning environment herself when she was a student and believes that for students to learn, it is necessary for them to replay her experience. Bright, enquiring students may pose a threat by asking questions that members of trained staff are unable to answer (Marson 1982). The consequence of this is that trained staff may distance themselves from that student. The student tends to become a scapegoat and perceived as a troublemaker, when in fact all she was doing was developing an understanding of individual care processes.

Ogier's (1981) study of ward sisters' influence upon nurse learners showed that students perceived positively those sisters who spent most time interacting with students. If you reflect on your own interactions between your students and other members of staff, it may help you to identify the actual amount of time you spend on this activity.

Orton (1981) and Fretwell (1982) in their studies of the ward learning climate found that the aspects students valued highly were:

- being treated kindly with understanding and staff who were willing to teach them

- being encouraged to ask questions without being made to feel foolish

- being made to feel important.

From these few examples, it can be seen that the practice learning climate has an influential part to play in creating an environment that is conductive to learning.

Activity 2.5.

Spend a few minutes reflecting on what you have just read. Then write down what you believe to be the key factors in creating a good learning climate.

Now examine the extent to which these can be found in your own learning environment.

The influence and the part played by practitioner-teachers in creating environments conducive to learning cannot be over-emphasised. Research shows that the charge nurse/ward sister is a key figure in creating such a climate. She also has a role-model influence. Danziger (1976) suggests that it is the observation of the model and not the interaction with him or her that is important for social learning to occur. Whilst the amount of teaching that the charge nurse/ward sister engages in may not be large, they may have a significant part to play in shaping and influencing the learning environment.

CONCLUSION

This chapter has examined the meaning of assessment and its application in identifying needs. It has explored the relationship between assessment of a learner within a teaching situation and the variables that influence the assessment process.

You have been encouraged to reflect on your own role as a practitioner-teacher.

Finally, the chapter introduced you to a number of concepts that relate both to you as a teacher and the assessment process, encouraging you to examine the theory underpinning assessment and enabling you to develop a greater awareness of your role as an assessor. We hope that it will have stimulated you to read more about assessment and will have helped you to realise the need for a reflective enquiring attitude toward your practice.

REFERENCES

Bligh D A (1972) *What's the Use of Lectures?* London: Penguin Books.

Bond C F (1982) Social Facilitation: a Self-presentation View. *Journal of Personality and Social Psychology*, **42**, 1042–1050.

Coates V E and Chambers M (1990) Developing a System of Student-nurse Profiling through Action Research. *Nurse Education Today*, **10**, 83–91.

Danziger K (1976) *Socialisation*. Penguin Books.

Fretwell J E (1982) *Ward Teaching and Learning: sister and the learning environment*. London: Royal College of Nursing.

Holloway P J, Hardwick J L, Morris J and Stout K B (1967) The Validity of Essay and Viva-Voce Examining Techniques, in Rowntree D (1987) *Assessing Students: How shall we know them?* London: Kogan Page.

Kelly E (1958) A Study of Consistent Discrepancies between Instructor Grades and Term-end Examination Grades. *Journal of Educational Psychology*, **49**, 328–334.

Kolb D A (1984) *Experiential Learning as the Science of Learning and Development*. New Jersey: Prentice Hall.

Kolb D A, Rubin I M and McIntyre J M (1971) *Organisational Psychology: an experiential approach*. New Jersey: Prentice Hall, in Boydell T (1976) *Experiential Learning*, Manchester monography.

Marshall M S (1960) Teaching without Grades, Corrallis, in Rowntree D (1987) *Assessing Students: How shall we know them?* London: Kogan Page.

Marson S M (1982) *Ward Teaching Skills—an investigation into the behaviour characteristics of effective ward staff*, unpublished M.Phil Thesis, Sheffield City Polytechnic.

Maslow A H (1987) *Motivation and Personality*. London: Harper and Row.

Ogier M (1981) *An Ideal Sister*. London: Royal College of Nursing.

Orton H O (1981) *Ward Learning Climate: a study of the role of the ward sister in relation to student nurse learning on the ward*. London: Royal College of Nursing.

Rowntree D (1987) *Assessing Students: How shall we know them?* London: Kogan Page.

Vernon (1933) and Wolff (1943) p.29, in Maslow A H (1987), *Motivation and Personality*. London: Harper and Row.

Wicklund R A and Duval S (1971) Opinion Change and Performance Facilitation as a Result of Objective Self-awareness. *Journal of Experimental Social Psychology*, **7**, 319–342.

Wright D (1970) *Handbook for the Assessment of Experiential Learning; Learning from Experience Trust*. London: Twentieth Century Press.

FURTHER READING

Bradshaw P L (1989) *Teaching and Assessing in Clinical Nursing Practice*, pp 160–174. London: Prentice Hall. This chapter offers you another angle on the assessment of clinical performance. It focuses on clinical assessment as it relates to the nurses', midwives' and health visitors' rules. It shows you how levels of competence can be identified and assessed.

Brookfield S D (1986) *Understanding and Facilitating Adult Learning*, pp 261–282. Milton Keynes: Open University Press. You will find this chapter helpful in describing evaluation as it relates to learning and this should enable you to differentiate between assessment and evaluation.

Dunn D (1984) Have you done my Report please, Sister? *Nursing Times*, 4(2), April 4, 56–59. You will find this article interesting as it addresses many of the issues professionals face daily. It focuses on behaviour and assessment techniques and the implications for nurse education and training.

Mackereth P (1989) An Investigation of the Developmental Influences on Nurses' Motivation for their Continuing Education. *Journal of Advanced Nursing*, 14, 776–787. This article focuses on the importance of continuing education and motivational factors associated with it. Whilst this article will enable you to reflect on aspects of nurse education at both pre- and post-registration, pages 778–779 will be of particular interest in relation to the section here on motivation.

Rae L (1985) *The Skills of Human Relations Training*, pp 16–29, 30–49, 211–232, 233–260. Aldershot: Gower Publishing. This is an excellent book for professionals involved in teaching and practice. There are aspects in every chapter that you will find valuable. The chapter on 'the skills of learning' you will find helpful as it addresses learning, preferences, barriers to learning and learning styles. The chapter on 'observing human behaviour' you will find useful in relation to observation and assessment. Again, the chapter 'On the job problem solving' explores the coaching concept. The other chapter you should read is the one on 'Assessing the effectiveness of training'.

Smith R (1986) Skills for the Teacher. *Senior Nurse*, 4(4), April, 21. This short article discusses the importance of teaching and its relationship to assessment and learning.

3
Planning for Teaching

Introduction

This chapter is designed to help you plan your teaching. It will explore what is being taught and a selection of methods which you may wish to employ in order to maximise learning. Some of you may be very experienced at using some of the strategies contained in this section, whilst others may be on unfamiliar territory. Indeed, there will be areas in which each of you is expert, particularly in matters relating to clinical practice. By working through this chapter and reflecting on your own expertise and strengths, your teaching will become more effective and efficient.

You will be introduced to a variety of methods which may be adopted or adapted to suit different situations. You will also have the opportunity to explore some of the newer concepts and systems introduced into nursing and midwifery education.

Within the chapter there will be opportunities to think about the student in terms of their individuality and how you as the teacher can respond to different demands made upon you; at the same time you will have the opportunity to reflect on your own needs as a teacher and indeed in some instances as a student.

Some of you will already be involved in Project 2000 courses (UKCC 1986) and therefore will have some experience of working with students undertaking this preparation for practice whilst on placement in the clinical areas; some of you will be preparing for the introduction of Project 2000, and yet others of you may be students on Project 2000 courses or on a post-registration Diploma or National Board teaching course. With this in mind, because of the nature of the different teaching requirements, it is important that levels of teaching and information are considered. The likelihood is that the teaching with which you have been involved, to a greater or lesser extent, will have been in the clinical area, and as such, the type of teaching would probably be directed towards assisting the student to acquire practical competence. In this chapter you will, as stated earlier, have the opportunity to explore different methods. It is not the intention that these methods be dealt with in great detail but rather that the key concepts will be included, together with a short description of the method, with suggestions for further reading.

The nursing and midwifery professions have for a long time valued the attributes of maturity and responsibility amongst their members. However, many of the educational programmes undertaken by students failed to respond to these characteristics. Recently there have been considerable advances in education, which have been made available to the general public, for example, access courses to nursing, open and distance learning packages and flexistudy courses. Also included in this are the courses provided and approved by the Training and Enterprise Councils (TECs). This has in many ways ensured that the particular needs of the adult as a student are met by offering a more flexible approach to learning. Nurses, whether they are undertaking pre- or post-registration courses have a right to this enlightened approach to their own education.

Activity 3.a.

At this point, before moving on, stop for a moment and think about your own experiences as a student.

Did you feel that those involved in your education treated you as an adult?

If you trained some time ago then you may have experienced situations similar to the following:

1. Your sessions in 'the School of Nursing' were timetabled with little reference to you as an individual and your own particular needs;

2. the style of teaching was determined by the teacher with little reference to the preferred learning style of the student;

3. teaching was teacher-centred, in that the topic being dealt with was decided by the teacher in relation to the syllabus, and the level at which it was taught was also decided by the teacher;

4. the teacher decided what the student should know;

5. objectives were set which had to be achieved by *all* students and the expected level of achievement was *pre-determined*.This was the same for both theoretical work and practical experience;

6. there was little flexibility in approach to teaching and learning.

You can probably think of many other similar instances but essentially the answer to the question 'Were you treated as an adult?' is 'no'.

However, you are now in a position to do something about it and ensure that your students do not experience a similar situation.

Activity 3.b.

What approaches do you feel are particularly pertinent to adult students? Jot your ideas down.

As you work through this chapter some of the ideas you have made a note of will be expanded upon and you may wish to add to your list, but to give you some idea of what your list might look like, here are some considerations for adult students:

- an open friendly approach

- recognition of the person as an individual

- acceptance of the person's strengths and weaknesses

- being non-judgemental and accepting the person for who he or she is

- seeking the person's ideas about their learning needs

- recognising the person's experience of life

- being aware of the individual's opinions and their personal values and beliefs and accepting these.

Notice that these points do not necessarily refer to *what* to teach but rather *how*. For some of you, lack of confidence in your own ability to undertake this part of your role is something you need to overcome. By working through this chapter some of the 'how' questions will be answered and certainly your confidence should be increased.

In chapter 1 of this book you were introduced to the part that you, as a practitioner, play in the educational process and the teaching element of your role, irrespective of your particular discipline. This overview should have given you a good insight into what teaching is about. Now we will take an in-depth look.

3.1. TEACHING—THE PROCESS

In its simplest form, teaching is the way in which one person brings about learning in another . . . a simple enough concept to grasp but teaching and learning are not inextricably linked.

Activity 3.1a.

Think about the following statement:

Teaching is not essential to learning

What does this imply to you?

Is it true?

Can you think of an example of where someone might learn without being taught in the clinical area?

This is not to say that teaching is unimportant or irrelevant . . . on the contrary, it is vital. The reason for posing this statement, and asking you to think about it, is that adults as students sometimes engage in more learning than is often acknowledged. Having said this, can such learning be classed as education?

According to Jarvis (1988), education can be defined as any planned series of incidents having a humanistic basis directed towards the participant's learning and understanding (page 27).

The acquisition of knowledge, skills and attitudes can be the result of study, experience or teaching and therefore could be construed as education.

During your own professional education, phrases such as formal and informal teaching have probably been heard.

Formal teaching
Could be described as a teacher/student interaction which has been planned in advance.

Informal teaching
A teaching/learning situation which arises spontaneously, i.e. a 'teachable moment'.

Activity 3.1b.

Stop for a moment and consider learning episodes from your own experience, either as a student or qualified practitioner, which you would class as either 'formal' or 'informal'. Having made your list, what do you consider to be the advantages and disadvantages of each approach? Finally, do you consider it to be both desirable and possible to develop an integrated approach with a balance of formal and informal methods, or should you choose one or the other?

One of the advantages of the 'formal' session is that both the teacher and student know what the encounter is designed to do.

An advantage of the informal method is that the learning opportunity is made extremely meaningful when the situation arises and could be a form of action learning.

Nurse education is usually a combination of the two methods. As a teacher the principles underlying both forms of teaching are the same.

At this point it may be relevant to look at some of the theories which have contributed to our understanding of teaching and learning. Of necessity these will be brief accounts and in no way are they intended to be thought of as the only ways in which teaching and learning can be approached. They are offered to illustrate approaches which you may wish to adopt. The order in which each is dealt with is not indicative of preference . . . the choice is yours.

3.1.1. THE HUMANISTIC APPROACH

This approach to teaching and learning centres particularly around the writings of Carl Rogers (1969, 1983), who is noted for his work in relation to counselling and psychotherapy. This approach is described as non-directive, and focuses on the human qualities of conveying warmth and empathy, in an attempt to encourage a greater understanding of self. It does not impose or direct the individual, but rather facilitates the learning process. Rogers holds the view that the individual has a natural propensity to learn and it is on this inner drive that this method relies. By acting as a facilitator to the process of learning you are encouraging the individual to learn that which they perceive as important and which will enhance or maintain their concept of self.

Facilitation is a process by which you enable the student to experience a variety of situations without dictating the terminal behaviour or directing the student.

Activity 3.1.1a.

Take time to consider the students in your area.

When the student first arrives in the area, how do you determine what he or she will learn?

How involved is the student in this decision?

Keep these notes handy for use later in the chapter.

By acting as a facilitator you are not taking control of the situation but rather working in partnership with the student in order (a) to identify what the student's own needs are, (b) to ensure that the student has the opportunity to undertake a variety of experiences and (c) to develop up to his/her level of achievement.

As a practitioner involved in this approach, you have to consider how learning will best be achieved and what your role in the process is. Listed below are some ideas for you to consider . . . you will probably think of more.

The student's learning will be enhanced when she is working in an environment where there is a climate of trust and where a non-threatening approach is adopted. Learning is on a shared basis, where there is mutual participation of both facilitator and student and this learning is brought about through experience. Since this approach relies on the inner drives, the intrinsic motivation of the student to learn, the student is encouraged to evaluate his/her own performance; indeed the student is seen as the prime innovator and evaluator of his/her own learning. The humanistic approach to education has received a good deal of attention in recent years, particularly in the area of psychiatry, where nurse teachers in mental health place great emphasis and value on the growth and development of students. From this approach grew the concept of 'experiential learning'.

Activity 3.1.1b.

What do you understand by the term experiential learning and what do you think its characteristics are?

Experiential Learning

The characteristics which consistently emerge from the theory and practice of experiential learning are as follows:

- the emphasis is on action;

- students are encouraged to reflect on their own experience;

- a clarifying approach is adopted by the facilitator;

- there is an accent on personal experience;

- human experience is valued as a source of learning

(Burnard 1990).

In many colleges of nursing and midwifery experiential strategies are now fairly common-place and are integrated into the curriculum. This non-directive approach to teaching and learning is of great relevence to people like yourself, working within the clinical areas, who are ideally situated to facilitate learning through experience.

Activity 3.1.1c.

Take time to consider your own work environment, focusing on what you have to offer the student in terms of experience available. Keep your responses for reference later in the chapter when we look at planning teaching.

Obviously this list will vary considerably depending on your area of work and the stage which the student is at, but to give you a couple of examples:

1. pre- and post-operative care of patients/clients undergoing surgery

2. care of the patient/client with intravenous infusion in situ

Your list will probably be more comprehensive.

Colleges of nursing and midwifery aim to equip students with the knowlege and skills to enable them to function within the clinical setting. However, it is fair to say that theory does not always precede practice. Within the educational process there is a place for both relating learned theory to practice and relating learned practice to the theory underpinning it. As stated earlier, practitioners are in a strong position to ensure appropriate learning in the clinical environment, since a good proportion of the student's time is spent in the practice area. It is therefore important that you are familiar with the curriculum model adopted within your College of Nursing and Midwifery.

What is a curriculum model? Burrel (1988) describes a curriculum model as an organised set of ideas or concepts, which displays in words or diagrams the essential features of the venture.

Activity 3.1.1d.

Make an appointment with the head of the curriculum planning team within your college (or if there is no specific team, get in touch with the head of pre-registration/post-registration studies depending on the type of student you have in your area) and discuss the curriculum model in use.

In your discussions you may wish to focus on:

1. the choice of model;

2. why the college selected the model they use;

3. an overview of the curriculum and how each part fits in to form the whole educational package for students;

4. how progression is demonstrated throughout the curriculum;

5. the curriculum model and how the philosophy underpinning it is put into practice;

6. whether the model in use fits in with the humanistic approach in the way it treats the student;

7. whether the model is a *product model* or a *process model* (see chapter 4 for a discussion of these terms).

In discussion there are likely to be other questions which will arise as a result of the information you get.

As a practitioner responsible for the educational experiences of the student on placement in your clinical area, you are in a position to control:

1. what is available in terms of experience

2. the quality of the experience available

3. the quantity of experience available

Activity 3.1.1e.

Back to your notes on the experiences you can offer students, which you compiled in Activity 3.1.1a

From this list identify those experiences which can only be experienced in your area of practice and those which could be offered elsewhere

You should now have a list of experiences which the student can *only* undertake in your area

Keep this safely, together with the earlier list

Rogers (1983) uses the word 'significant' to describe the kind of learning which is pervasive and can make a difference to both attitudes and behaviour. Nursing is traditionally sympathetic to the spirit of this humanistic approach, since learning is seen as an emotional experience as well as a cognitive one. In the last two decades a good deal of research was undertaken in relation to the student in the clinical area and the provision of a good learning climate. Attention was also drawn to the significance of the role of the ward sister in the socialisation process of students whilst on placement in the clinical areas (see Orton 1981, Ogier 1982, 1986 and Gott 1983, 1984).

Activity 3.1.1f.

Locate within your college of nursing and/or midwifery a copy of the following articles, which you should find interesting. They are both related to the socialisation process of students in relation to the ward learning climate.

Sheahan J (1978) Ward Sister: Manager, Nurse or Teacher? *Nursing Mirror*, 135, pp 18–21

Fretwell J E (1980) An Enquiry into the Ward Learning Environment. Occasional Paper, *Nursing Times*, 76(16), pp 69–75

Although the article by Sheahan is quite old, it is still worth reading and should be filed with the back issues of the *Nursing Mirror* (now taken over by the *Nursing Times*).

Experiential learning is an appropriate method to be adopted in the clinical setting. However, for it to be effective all the participants in the process must be fully involved.

In order to ensure the viability of this approach you need to be aware of the role of the teacher in the process. Rogers (1983) gives guidelines for facilitators in the learning process. Briefly, the facilitator should:

1. *Show concern wih establishing a climate of trust*

Activity 3.1.1g.

What do you consider to be the important points in order to establish trust?

Having given this some thought you may have come up with points such as:

1. honesty
2. being a real person and not putting up a front
3. personal contact with the student
4. accepting the student as a person
5. giving the student responsibility
6. accepting the student's opinions
7. awareness of the student's feelings

Together with any others which you think are important.

2. *Identify the learning needs of individual students*

Activity 3.1.1h.

Refer to your list of experiences available to students whilst in your area of practice.

How will you set about catering for the needs of individual students?

Points you may wish to consider in relation to this activity are the need to:

continued on next page

continued

1. ascertain the student's level of competence

2. find out the student's areas of interest

3. discuss the overall intention of the experience

4. discuss with the student what their personal expectations are from the experience.

These are just a few points to get you started. You may wish to review again the chapter related to assessing learning needs (chapter 2).

Activity 3.1.1i.

This activity is closely associated with the preceding one but asks you to think about the mechanisms you will adopt to ensure that the student's needs are met.

Here are a few ideas to get you started:

1. identify resources available

2. pool the expertise of the staff

3. discuss the experiences available with all concerned.

3. *Increase student motivation in achieving that which is significant to her* Although it was stated earlier in this chapter that this approach to teaching and learning relies on the inner drives of the student to learn, these can be enhanced by external motivators. This refers to strategies you might employ to encourage the student in her quest for knowledge and experience. For example:

1. showing an interest in the student as both a person and as a learner

2. giving praise

3. providing reassurance that she is developing appropriately as a practitioner of the future

4. ensuring that the student is aware of the level of performance expected

5. offering constructive criticism

6. suggesting explanations where appropriate

4. *Ensure the availability of and access to a wide range of experiences*

You have already moved quite a long way towards meeting this in the activities you have undertaken, in relation to identifying what experiences are available in your area of practice.

5. *Act as a resource*

Acting as a resource does not imply that you have to be a 'fount of all knowledge', indeed this would be impossible to achieve. What is does mean is that if you don't know, you can locate someone who can help. Essentially, by acting as a resource, you are able to direct the student to the most appropriate sources of information. Do not forget that when you have to say 'I don't know' you can use this as a valuable learning opportunity to learn alongside your student.

6. *Accept the student as a person*

On the face of it this seems fairly easy, but there will be some students with whom you will not find it easy to relate. They have the same rights to education in your area as any other student, so there are times when you have to put aside your own feelings and prejudices. This, of course, works both ways; the student has the obligation to act in the same way and accept you as a person.

7. *Share his/her own thoughts and feelings*

This means being open and honest; making it clear that you care about the student and her professional development and also that you care for the student as a person. It also includes sharing your thoughts and feelings about situations which may be encountered by the student and yourself, in which the student may feel inadequate or distressed. It is important that students know that these are situations in which we all experience problems or painful feelings, and sharing them can boost the students' confidence.

8. *Recognise conflict or tensions which may arise and use these as a learning experience*
Situations can arise within the work environment which provoke anger or resentment and if not dealt with, this can inhibit students' progress.

By exploring the situation with the student you can turn what may be a counterproductive situation into a very productive *learning* situation. For example: take a situation where a patient has exhibited aggressive behaviour. These sorts of outbursts cause tension and sometimes students cannot come to terms with their own feelings following such an incident. By exploring this with the student you can put things into perspective and allay some of the anxieties the student may have.

9. *Reflect and accept his/her own strengths and weaknesses*
This is really quite difficult and requires you to be honest with yourself. It may be just as hard to acknowledge strengths as it is to explore less strong areas.

Activity 3.1.1j.

What are your good points? (Not just in relation to teaching or to your practice, but generally.) Are you, for example, punctual, a loyal friend, generous?

What areas do you need to improve? (For instance, are you untidy, impatient in areas where you lack understanding, tending to assume control in relationships?)

Take some time to think about this one.

Having identified your strengths remember that you need to keep these to the forefront of your mind and nurture them—don't just file them in your memory. Strengths should be *used* just as areas in need of improvement need working on.

Summary of the humanistic approach

Phase one
The initial phase occurs when the student's learning needs are identified through shared activities, between you as the teacher and the student as the taught. Using this information, both you and the student plan the

learning experience. The student is perceived as the *prime-innovator* of his/her own learning needs, to ensure that the required level of achievement is attained. Account is taken of the student's perception of what is important to her.

Phase two
This is an interactive phase, i.e. it encompasses the experience which the student is undergoing in order to learn. This is a shared exploration of the experience between you and the student. When adopting this approach to teaching and learning, it is not possible to predetermine the 'product' at the end of the experience, since different experiences will have a different meaning for and effect on individual students, who will each react differently to the situation. This is where knowing your student as an individual is important. It is not necessarily *what* the student learns that is of prime importance, but the *process* of learning and how significant that learning is to the student together with the contribution it makes to the student's development.

Phase three
This consists of the evaluative process, with the student as the prime evaluator of her development. Those involved in the experience are asked to add their perceptions of the student's progress in order to give an overall picture and to identify areas where more development is required.

3.1.2. THE EXPERIENTIAL APPROACH

This approach to teaching and learning was first explored by Steinaker and Bell (1979) who claimed to offer a 'Gestalt Taxonomy' that would provide a framework for understanding, planning and evaluating the meaning of a **Total experience**. They refer to the much used cognitive, affective and psychomotor domains as useful curriculum planning tools, but argued that because each dealt with only one aspect of human interaction within an experience, their use is limited. Because the student understands the way in which a skill is performed and may indeed be able to explain it, it does not mean that the student can perform that skill. So as you can see, there is not always obvious correlation between cognitive and psychomotor activity.

The experiential taxonomy explicitly reveals learning objectives and principles; student and teacher strategies and evaluation techniques; and has the potential to eliminate the discrepancy between theory and practice, whilst giving prominence to attitudinal and interpersonal skills. As with the other commonly described taxonomies (Bloom 1964, Krathwohl 1968 and Simpson 1966), the experiential taxonomy can demonstrate progression, in terms of level of development, and in this sense the experiential taxonomy is a useful educational tool; it not only includes educationally planned and defined experiences but also incorporates everyday experience.

The experiential taxonomy is divided into five categories which demonstrate its progressive nature. Later in this book we will look at a possible way in which this taxonomy could be used in the teaching of models of practice in nursing and midwifery.

Categories of the experiential taxonomy
1. **Exposure**: normally refers to the initial encounter with an experience and the students' awareness of that experience.

2. **Participation**: assumes the student accepts exposure to the experience and is willing to proceed to overt/covert participation.

3. **Identification**: the student makes a choice to identify with certain aspects of the experience.

4. **Internalisation**: goes beyond intellectual and emotional acceptance and becomes a new way of perceiving and being.

5. **Dissemination**: the highest level of knowledge and skill in terms of the experiential taxonomy. The student finishes as a proficient new role model, capable of critical appraisal.

The two terms experiential taxonomy and experiential learning are not necessarily synonymous. A curriculum built on the experiential taxonomy can utilise learning methods other than, or in addition to, experiential learning.

The perception of many teachers is that experiential learning is confined to **role play, gaming** and **simulation**. This was reinforced by Bevis (1982) when she described the first function of the teacher as providing a structure for the successful playing of the game, when utilising experiential learning techniques. The experiential taxonomy is much more than a teaching and learning strategy. The underlying assumption is that for learning to take place, the student has to undergo the experience. If this is accepted, the taxonomy is seen as a series of stages taking the student from the initial exposure through to its ultimate incorporation into the student's observable behaviour. In effect this experience could be real or simulated or it may be neither. A formal lecture, in this sense, would be seen as a valuable learning experience as indeed would be reading this book!

In essence, it is a deceptively simple yet psychologically sound instrument. Although the taxonomy was developed for use in general education and for the in-service training of teachers, its application can be much wider. This can be seen from the number of colleges of nursing and midwifery which have adopted this approach to education for both pre and post-registration courses. A further application can be seen in a series of articles in *Senior Nurse* in which this taxonomy has been applied to the clinical setting (see Further Reading for details).

3.1.3. THE THEORY OF ANDRAGOGY AND PEDAGOGY

The term andragogy refers to 'the art and science of helping adults to learn', whereas pedagogy is 'the art and science of teaching children' (Knowles 1970, 1973).

Activity 3.1.3a.

What do you consider to be the main differences between teaching children and helping adults to learn?

The two models, i.e. pedagogy and andragogy, should not be seen as being in opposition but rather as running in parallel and either can be equally appropriate, depending on circumstances. Each model makes a different assumption about the individual, based on five dimensions:

1. concept of the student

2. role of the student's experience

3. the student's readiness to learn

4. the student's orientation to learning

5. the student's motivation to learn.

Pedagogy

First let us examine the assumptions with a pedagogical approach:

1. **Concept of the student**:   the student is dependent on the teacher who controls and makes the major decisions regarding what the student learns.

2. **Role of the student's experience**:   most of this experience is of little use as the basis for learning. The pedagogical approach is

reliant on the transmission mode for teaching, i.e. telling the student.

3. **The student's readiness to learn**:   in this approach, the readiness to learn tends to be age-related or dependent on the biological stage of development.

4. **The student's orientation to learning**:   in this approach it is, in the main, subject-centred.

5. **The student's motivation to learn**:   tends to be from external pressures, e.g. parental, or teachers stressing the importance of education.

Andragogy

The **assumptions** that are made within this approach, using the five dimensions are:

1. **Concept of the student**:   tends to be more self-directed, with the student taking on board the responsibility for their own learning.

2. **The role of the student's experience**:   the individual's experience is of greater quantity (although varying quality) compared to that of children; it includes life experiences and experience of the different roles of adulthood, for example, parenthood, employee, student of further or higher education.

3. **The student's readiness to learn**:   this tends to be based on needs related to what the individual wants to know or needs to know in order to be able to do things.

4. **The student's orientation to learning**:   tends to be centred round life experiences rather than subject-based. The student needs the skills and knowledge to be able to identify and solve problems.

5. **The student's motivation**:   mainly intrinsic, with the student's need for self-esteem and self-worth as the major driving forces; this is confirmed by external motivators such as recognition, respect and feedback relating to learning development.

Knowles (1984) asserts that students move from dependence to independence during their maturation. Benner (1984) reaffirmed this in her study 'From Novice to Expert', focusing on the development of the student nurse. In the early stages of career development, the student is very dependent on the qualified practitioner for help and guidance, but through experience and appropriate skill acquisition she become an independent, advanced and expert practitioner.

Activity 3.1.3b.

Consider your own professional progress and development to date.

After gaining experience in one area of practice and moving on to another area, how confident did you feel?

What support mechanisms were available to help you through this period?

This principle of moving from dependence to independence has been expressed in the *Post-registration Education and Practice Project Report* (PREPP) (UKCC 1990).

Activity 3.1.3c.

Locate a copy of the PREPP Report (UKCC 1990) and have a look at the first two recommendations. They are elaborated in sections 4.4 and 4.10.

What are their implications for you personally?

These two recommendations are statements of good practice and examine the support required for the newly qualified practitioner, suggesting a mechanism for providing this support.

Activity 3.1.3d.

Take time to consider the support you got.

Did it match the recommended support?

Now consider whether this support should only be available to newly qualified practitioners or should it be extended to include those who are changing roles?

In essence, support of this kind should be available to everyone who is making a transition; for when qualified practitioners move to new areas of practice they are, in fact, moving back into the novice phase.

Activity 3.1.3e.

Refer back to the differences highlighted by Knowles (1984) in relation to the learning process for adults and think about the implications for you, as a teacher-practitioner involved in the educational process of adults, whether they are:

- colleagues
- other professionals
- patients/clients
- relatives.

Write down what you consider to be important factors in the process of teaching adults in your clinical area.

Your thoughts may fall under headings like those that follow:

Self-direction
- Students should be given responsibility for their own learning, and may, for example, be directed towards open and distance learning materials.

- Students are partners with the teacher in negotiating the learning experience. Indeed, they may together develop a learning contract where the ground-rules for their relationship are delineated.

- The teacher should not impose what she/he thinks the student needs to learn.

Experience
- The student should be accepted as an adult, and the life experiences the student has undergone should be used and adapted to enhance learning in the current situation.

- The teacher-practitioner should provide access to a wide range of experiences and should help the student to learn from an experience.

Readiness
The teacher-practitioner needs to:

- encourage development of the student's self-awareness, using positive feedback and constructive criticism and so build the student's self-confidence.
- respect the student as an individual with her own values/beliefs and opinions
- act as a partner in the learning process
- offer support to the student who may or may not accept it; nevertheless, it should be made clear that the support is on offer.

Orientation
- The teacher-practitioner is responsible for ensuring that the experience is realistic and relevant to the student
- She/he should take account of the individuality of each student and guide and support as required.

Motivation
It is encumbent upon the teacher-practitioner to:

- ensure that the learning meets the individual need of each student
- recognise the students' strengths and areas where they are less proficient and confident.

This list is not intended to be exhaustive, but it gives you some indication of the approach that is inherent within andragogy. Adults can bring to the learning situation a variety of life experiences which can be used as a valuable resource. For example, the student may have cared for a sick relative and had to deal with the support services and can help patients/clients with first-hand information. All learning is important and by adopting experiential methods these valuable resources can be tapped in helping students to grasp new situations.

An andragogical approach expresses the idea that adults learn when they need to know or to do, in order to be able to function more effectively or efficiently.

You are a good example in having decided that, in order to perform your role more effectively, you need to know more about teaching and so you have set about studying this book.

3.1.4.   BEHAVIOURAL APPROACHES

Perhaps the most significant contribution made to the behavioural psychology of learning is that of Skinner. He developed the theory of **operant conditioning** which formed the basis for **programmed learning**, which was very popular in the 1960s. (Programmed learning could be seen as the forerunner to computer-assisted learning (CAL) but the learning materials were text-based rather than on computer.) Some of you who trained during this period may have first-hand experience of this approach.

Skinner (1968) suggested that teaching is the arrangement of reinforcements under which students learn, i.e. that learning is the acquisition of new behaviours through a system of reward and punishment. To give you an example of this system which is not related to nursing, undertake the next activity.

Activity 3.1.4a.

Think back to your childhood days, or indeed, to times bringing up your own family when good behaviour was rewarded favourably and bad behaviour resulted in some form of punishment.

This system of reward and punishment was also adopted in clinical practice, particularly in psychiatry, with the introduction of token economy schemes and behaviour modification programmes. In token economy schemes clients were rewarded with a 'token' for exhibiting appropriate behaviour and this 'token' was acted as a form of currency, which the client could exchange for cigarettes, etc.

This approach to teaching and learning could be referred to as 'training', the emphasis of which is clearly on an overt change in behaviour as a result of learning and it had a significant impact on nurse education.

When employing this system of teaching and learning, the student's development is predetermined by the acquisition of set aims and objectives, which are written in terms of changes in behaviour which are observable and measurable. It may be an appropriate point to stop and consider what aims and objectives are.

Aims and objectives in teaching
An aim is an overall statement of what the learner must be able to do at the end of a given period of instruction or experience.

For example, 'at the end of the course of instruction the learner must be able to drive a car safely and correctly at all times in all conditions.' In order to be able to achieve that aim there are certain things that the learner must be able to do and some of these must be taught in a specific and critical order. Because there needs to be a logical progression and so that continuity can be maintained, it is essential that these things must be written down and the teacher must be able to measure whether learning has taken place so that the student can move on to the next step.

These steps (or stepping stones) are called educational objectives.

Educational objectives
must be

- specific

- observable and measurable by an observer

- realistic

- consistent for *all* learners

- continuously evaluated.

Teaching and experience are geared to meeting such objectives.

An example of objectives, related to learning to drive, might be as follows:

- Certain criteria must be met before the person is eligible to learn to drive. For example: age, health, physical characteristics.

- before the car even moves the learner must be able to:
  (a) see out of the windscreen and see into the rear view mirror when sitting in the driving position,
  (b) reach the pedals (with both feet) whilst sitting in the driving seat and maintaining vision,
  (c) reach the gear lever wtih the left hand whilst maintaining vision and foot control,
  (d) demonstrate an ability to distinguish between the accelerator pedal, the foot brake and the clutch without the use of vision,
  (e) demonstrate an ability to co-ordinate the use of the left and right hands relating to the steering wheel and the gear lever (and so on).

Do you see how objectives detail the steps of the skill sequentially and how each starts with a verb?

For example:

The aim of psychiatric nurse training
The aim is to produce an individual with knowledge, skill and compassion, who can make a valuable contribution to the care of the psychiatrically ill person in hospital or the community.

The aim of the introductory course
The aim of the introductory course is to orientate the new student to the College of Nursing and the Mental Health Unit.

It is intended to introduce the student to the concepts of caring for the mentally ill client/patient and to ensure that the student has sufficient information for them to participate in, and appreciate, some of the care and treatment which they will observe during their first experience in the clinical areas.

Some of the objectives of the introductory course might be to:

- discuss the role of the Registered Mental Nurse and their own role in relation to the therapeutic team and patients.

- itemise the various health authority policies as they apply to nursing in the Mental Health Unit, and be able to demonstrate an ability to carry out correctly the desired behaviour in the event of fire, violence and missing patient/client.

- examine the implications of the Mental Health Act and identify the most important sections in relation to their present stage in training.

- describe the links which exist between the Mental Health Unit and the Community and Social Services.

Reasons for using aims and objectives
- They cause the teacher to focus on exactly what it is that they want the learner to achieve,

- they help to ensure continuity and consistency in teaching and training,

- they set minimum acceptable standards of performance,

- they allow other people, including the students, to see what is required,

- they clarify what is to be taught, what is essential and how topics should be taught.

Activity 3.1.4b.

As a teacher-practitioner, how would you assess whether a student was meeting his or her objectives in a clinical placement?

Here are one or two suggestions:

— unbiased observation, watching the student at work
— by setting written essays on a relevant topic
— asking the students to demonstrate the skill in question
— monitoring the improvement in skill performance
— discussing with the students the theory underlying the skill

As students gain fulfilment from making objectives, this may well result in lowering of sickness rates, lowering of absence rates and increased stability in the ward team.

Gibson (1980) believes that the impact of behavioural objectives should not be underestimated.

Activity 3.1.4c.

We have said that a behavioural approach to learning depends on its success on reinforcement.

What do you think are the likely rewards to which an adult may respond?

Your list may include:

(a) praise
(b) constructive criticism
(c) recognition of self as well as strengths
(d) anything that might increase self-esteem and self-worth.

Nowadays the influence of behaviourism in nurse education is receding. Davies (1976) suggests that behavioural objectives serve three broad areas. They serve as guides:

1. for curriculum planning and teaching
2. to learning
3. for teacher and student evaluation.

Few nurse teachers would adopt a purely behavioural model by solely applying behavioural objectives when preparing teaching programmes. For, in nurse education, we are concerned with the development of the individual into a competent nurse, which involves considerably more than changes in behaviour patterns. You, as a teacher-practitioner in the clinical area, are probably experienced in setting objectives—not necessarily for teaching but rather for patient/client care. However, the principles are the same:

1. you identify what the problem is
2. what you can do about it
3. what the desired end result (outcome) should be.

The same applies to education:

1. you identify what the student needs in terms of experience
2. what you can offer
3. what the desired level of achivement should be.

It might be relevant at this point to look at the three areas or domains in which the student is to develop. These are:

The Cognitive Domain—Bloom (1964)
The Affective Domain—Krathwohl (1968)
The Psychomotor Domain—Simpson (1966)

The Cognitive Domain is concerned with the development of the student's intellectual skills. Within this domain there are varying levels which can be identified and measured in terms of development of intellectual skills.
The Affective Domain is concerned with the student's development of attitudes, values and beliefs. The levels of this domain demonstrate progression, but are more difficult to determine.

The Psychomotor Domain is concerned with the development of motor skills.

Gagne (1983) suggested that learning consists of sequential stages founded on prerequisite abilities or intellectual skills. This principle has relevance to clinical education in the practice setting. When students come to your clinical area for experience you have knowledge of:

1.   their stage in development, i.e. 1st, 2nd, 3rd year, and based on this and your assessment of their prior knowledge and experience, you plan their experience.

2.   what you expect the student to be able to do and the appropriate level of performance.

During the experience, when working with the student, you guide the student through a sequence from basic to more skilled performance.

Gagne stressed the importance of giving students immediate feedback related to their performance. As a supervisor you may find that students respond to limited criticism and periodic praise. It is important to remember that praise and criticism should be well balanced, in that, if you praise students all the time, it becomes meaningless; similarly if you criticise all the time, they become disheartened and come to feel that whatever they do they will never satisfy you.

Activity 3.1.4d.

Look back on the way in which you give students feedback on their performance. This is followed up in the next Activity.

It is likely that if you highlight the positive aspects of their performance first, they will be more responsive to the constructive criticism!

Finally, it is important that the student's contribution to the work of the caring team is recognised. A simple 'thank you' at the end of a busy day will go a long way towards making the student feel a valued member of the team and will enhance learning.

To Summarise the Behavioural Approach

Phase one
During this initial phase, time is spent with the student to ascertain his or

her learning needs, matching them to the experience you can offer. Discussion with the student about the experience, what you expect and the level of performance you require is important in setting the scene and giving the student direction. At this point you should explain to the student what is expected of them at the end of the experience, i.e. the explicit terminal behaviour. You would also explain how you will act to ensure the student's success.

Phase two
Consists of working with the student during the experience and observing their behaviour in the work situation. It is important during this phase that appropriate praise, criticism and feedback are given. You should identify the changes in the student's performance in moving towards the desired terminal behaviour. Some way through the experience, the terminal objectives should be reviewed with the student and feedback given as to how she is progressing. At this point you may highlight strengths and areas where improvement is necessary and together identify appropriate strategies to enable the student to succeed.

Phase three
This phase is concerned with establishing whether the student has achieved the predetermined objectives. These objectives and the level at which they are achieved are recorded. Where a student has not achieved an appropriate level, teaching continues.

This approach is of great value in skills training and so it is relevant at this point to consider skill acquisition.

Skill Acquisition

Activity 3.1.4f.

Select a skill which you teach to students regularly, for example, giving an injection, bathing a baby.

Read through this short section and then apply what you have read to teaching the skill.

Motor skills (i.e. being able to do things) are an extremely important aspect of the practice of nursing and midwifery. However, in practice we need to integrate the doing with knowledge about how and why things are done in that way, and an ability to interpret the results of performing the skill and so we refer to them as **psychomotor skills**. Motor skills are concerned with movement and a skilled person (practitioner) exhibits certain characteristics that a novice (student) does not yet possess.

Learning motor skills, unlike other forms of learning, requires practice, which consists of repetition under specific conditions. There are no obvious stages in this process, however, Fitts and Posner (1967) suggest three phases:

The Cognitive Phase

The Associative Phase

The Autonomous Phase

Refer to the skill that you have selected.
The Cognitive Phase.   This is concerned with learning the procedure. The more complex the skill the more time this will take. What knowledge does the student need in order to be able to undertake the skill?
The Associative Phase.   The learning is taking on characteristics of skilled performance and there is less 'fumbling'. The skill is 'raw' but complete, and the movement between the steps of the skill are becoming smoother.
The Autonomous Phase.   The skill becomes automatic.

The method you choose depends on the skill you are teaching. For example, fairly simple tasks are better learned in one session with periods of practice; more complex skills are better learned over a period of time, to avoid boredom, loss of attention and in some instances fatigue.

Activity 3.1.4g.

Reflect a moment on the range of skills that you teach. As you do so, decide whether you would put them into simple or complex categories.

At all times during this learning period, feedback to the student on his/her performance is essential. We have already established that immediate feedback is essential so that the student is aware of areas in which she is performing appropriately and those where more practice is required.

Activity 3.1.4i.

You may at this point wish to discuss with your colleagues in both clinical areas and the College of Nursing/Midwifery how they give feedback and think how you can improve.

We have so far established that teaching is one of the important functions of the practitioner and that it is a major nursing responsibility. Teaching in nursing or midwifery is an action-orientated, theoretically-based process. All qualified practitioners are obliged to teach and this is clearly stated in the Code of Professional Conduct (UKCC 1984):

'In the context of the individual's own knowledge, experience and sphere of authority, to assist peers and subordinates to develop a professional competence in accordance with their needs.'

The way in which you approach your 'teaching' is up to you. A good deal is done informally as you perform your clinical role. Remember that whatever teaching you do has a direct effect on patient care. By taking the time to plan your teaching logically, standards of care can be improved.

3.2.   TEACHING METHODS

This section of the chapter is designed to increase your awareness of the variety of methods which you can employ. By taking the time to explore the different methods, your ability to select methods appropriate to your needs will be enhanced.

As a student you will no doubt have experienced a variety of teaching methods. Some you will have enjoyed more than others.

Activity 3.2a.

Take time to reflect on your time as a student and some of the teaching methods you experienced

Which did you enjoy most/least and why?

There is an old adage which is well known to teachers:

'Tell 'em what you're going to tell 'em,
Then tell 'em,
Then tell 'em what you've just told 'em.

This is really the basis of planning teaching whatever the method you choose.

The principle can be applied to other situations. Next time you have the opportunity to view one of the old Hollywood-style slapstick comedies with 'the custard pie in the face' routine, watch carefully the sequence of events:

1. The 'deliverer' of the custard pie indicates what is going to happen, i.e. he is going to let the 'receiver' have it in the face!
    (Tell 'em what you're going to tell 'em)

2. 'The deliverer' delivers said custard pie to 'recipient'.
    (Then tell 'em)

3. 'The deliverer' holds empty plate and indicates content on 'receiver's' face and laughs.
    (Tell 'em what you've just told 'em!)

When considering your teaching, using the adage as a guide you need to plan the introduction, the development and the conclusion.

Introduction: this includes signposting for the student what the session is intended to cover. It also includes ascertaining the existing level of student attainment, and information on the method you are going to use. **Development**, i.e. the meat in the sandwich, involves working through your sequencing of information, etc.; giving feedback where relevant, and providing opportunities for practice. Throughout this section of teaching, the teacher should constantly check the learner's level of understanding.

The conclusion summarises the main points and uses them to draw the heads together, showing how the learning can be applied in future situations.

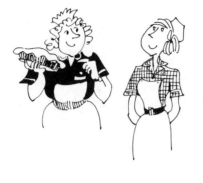

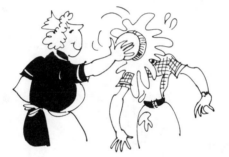

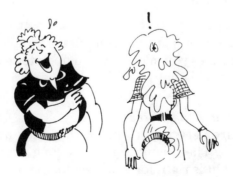

Although you will not always have the opportunity to draw up a formal teaching plan for a teaching session with notes, you should nevertheless allow yourself the time to focus on:

What do I want to teach?
— knowledge?

— a skill?

— a feeling?

— an attitude?

Why do I want to teach this?
— to give new knowlege?

— build on to previous knowledge?

— consolidate knowledge?

How shall I teach it?
— talk?

— show?

— supervise?

Do I need resources?
— paper?

— flip-chart?

— models?

— diagrams?

— overhead projector?

— books?

— patient or client?

You would be wise to prepare teaching notes for every session you under-take, although at times you may be called upon to teach something at such short notice that this is not possible.

Preparation of teaching notes
Teaching notes are very important, in that they act as a prompt in the teaching situation. There is no right or wrong way to prepare the notes you use, you do what is right for you, developing notes with which you feel comfortable. These notes, however, are best kept simple. Long essay-type notes tend to be confusing and difficult to follow in the teaching situation. Here are a few tips you may wish to follow:

1. Keep the notes brief and well spaced.

2. Use a highlighter pen to emphasise the main points so that when you glance down at them, they are clearly visible.

3. Number your pages and staple them together so that you do not risk them getting out of sequence if you drop them!

4. Consider using index cards which can be stored easily.

5. Update them regularly.

Let us go back to your reflections on the teaching methods you have experienced. Some will be included in the following descriptions and some of the methods described may be new to you. Sometimes you are teaching without really being aware of it; for example, a student will learn by watching how you behave and give care; how you manage your clinical area and how you supervise learners. Marson (1982) and Ogier and Barnett (1986) highlighted the importance of the role model in the student's learning process. An important facet of the student's development is the formation of appropriate attitudes, which may take time to describe or explain, but which can be quickly demonstrated by your every word and action (Bandura 1977).

3.2.1. Role Modelling

From this brief introduction, you can see that one method of enabling students to develop into advanced practitioners is by example. As an experienced practitioner you act as a key role model for junior staff and students.

All practitioners involved in the educative process transmit attitudes/values without consciously setting out to do so. This is part of what is known as the 'hidden curriculum'. It is a very important aspect of education and you need to be aware of it.

Activity 3.2.1a.

Reflect on the time when you were a student and identify a really good teacher with whom you were involved. What was it that made him/her a good teacher and in what ways would you like to be like him/her?

Role models such as those you have considered are remembered because of certain skills or attributes which seemed to you to be important as a nurse. It may be one individual or a collection of attributes from a variety of people with whom you came into contact.

Activity 3.2.1b.

In Activity 3.1.3c. you were asked to look at the first two recommendations of the PREPP Report (UKCC 1990).

Look again now at recommendation 2 in section 4.10. of the report

Visit your own College of Nursing and Midwifery and find out what mentorship or midwifery preceptorship schemes are in operation.

Now stop and think for a moment about the qualities you think are important in preceptors/mentors.

The role model within the culture of nursing has a powerful influence in the socialisation process. (The process of socialisation is discussed further in chapter 4.) Sheahan (1978) and Fretwell (1980) refer particularly to the role of the Ward Sister in this process, but all who come into contact with students have an effect to a greater or lesser degree. Social or observational learning occurs when one person learns something by observing another doing it—in other words learning takes place by modelling (Bandura 1977). Remember that this was discussed in chapter 1.

Whilst working alongside students in the clinical area, as well as setting examples of appropriate professional behaviour, you are required to pass on to the student certain psychomotor skills, by demonstrating the correct methods.

3.2.2. Demonstration

This can be defined as a visual explanation of facts, concepts and procedures, the purpose of which is to show the student how and why we perform the skill.

As an experienced practitioner you are, no doubt, an expert at the skills frequently encountered within your own clinical area. Can you remember what it was like when you first tried to perform a skill and did not have the confidence you now have when required to undertake something new?

In an earlier part of this chapter we explored briefly the theory of skills acquisition.

Activity 3.2.2a.

Consider the characteristics of a skilled performance.
What qualities do you have which you consider make you a good role model?

What aspects would you improve?

Within nursing and midwifery education not all motor skills need to be learned from scratch, since many of the component skills have already been mastered. It is therefore important to consider the entry behaviour, i.e. the knowledge, skills and attitudes which students bring to the learning situation.

Teaching a psychomotor skill

This involves the same principles as any other form of teaching. In the past many skills were taught in practice rooms within schools of nursing and midwifery, which were intended to simulate the ward environment. This practice has now been superseded by teaching these skills in the clinical area, which is the most appropriate place for the student to learn and practice. This, of course, does not apply to all practical skills, since it is important that certain skills are taught prior to the students working in the clinical areas. Simulation is not without problems and some students have difficulty in transferring what they are taught in the college to the clinical setting (Wong 1979).

Activity 3.2.2b.

Take time to consider those skills which you think should be taught in the college and those which are best taught in the clinical areas.

Give reasons for your choice.

Here are a couple of suggestions to help you with your choice.

1. Lifting

When students start to work in the clinical area, one of the skills required of them is that of lifting and moving patients/clients. It is important for the safety of all concerned that the student has had the opportunity to acquire knowledge about the procedure of lifting and has had the chance to practice under strict supervision. The skills can then be put into practice in the clinical area, and the risk of injury to the student, patient/client and teacher are minimised.

2. Resuscitation

Practice of this potentially life-saving procedure is normally undertaken using a resuscitation mannequin. This helps the students to familiarise themselves with the sequence of events and to practise the techniques involved away from the atmosphere of crisis that prevails in the 'real' situation.

Learning a skill takes time and this will vary, depending on the student and the compexity of the skill being taught. There are times when you are required to teach both students and patients/clients similar skills.

Activity 3.2.2c.

How would your approach differ between teaching a student and teaching a patient/client a similar skill?

When planning to teach a motor skill, the level at which the student must learn the skill has to be taken into consideration.

Activity 3.2.2d.

Take a few moments to think about the characteristics of a skilled performance, and list them. Your list may look something like this:

- It is **accurate**—that is, it is executed with precision.

- It is **efficient**: in other words it is economical in terms of effort expended, and the cost of equipment.

- It is **well-timed** with logical steps in the proper sequential order.

- It is **consistent** in its performance.

- It is conducted **swiftly** and with confidence.

- It is **adaptable**—the performer should be able to adapt the underlying principles to meet the needs of any patient/client.

- It is performed with **sensitivity**, the skilled practitioner obtaining the maximum information from the cues given by the client (e.g. regarding discomfort, anxiety) and being able to take appropriate actions to avoid unnecessary distress.

- **Anticipation** is evident, allowing a quick and appropriate response to any eventuality.

Teaching psychomotor skills requires provision of information and the opportunity for practice under supervision.

Activity 3.2.2e.

Think about a procedure you teach on a regular basis in your clinical area. How do you plan your teaching?

When you prepare to teach a skill you need to look at the whole of the skill and break it down into its component parts and then put it into a logical sequence. If you imagine you are teaching this to someone who knows nothing about it, you can then determine at which point in the sequence different students are able to enter, dependent on their entry behaviour.

3.2.3. Lectures

The term lecture is applied to a particular type of educational encounter, with the teacher doing most of the talking and the students listening. The term may be used to indicate a lesson, although lessons are usually considered to be less formal and consistent and more of a two-way interaction. Lectures can be a valuable learning method.

Table 3.1. Advantages and disadvantages of the lecture method.

Advantages	Disadvantages
Efficiency: 1 teacher: large number of students Well-presented lectures may motivate students New knowledge can be presented which is not generally available in text books Good for introducing new topics Useful for giving framework on which students can build or scene-setting	Students' attention may waver Students are largely passive Does not cater for individual needs Lecture environment may not be conducive to learning for some. Little opportunity to explore, question and analyse.

Numerous studies have been conducted on the advantages and disadvantages of lecturing (see Bligh 1972, Beard et al 1978 and Brown 1978). Their results can be summarised in Table 3.1.

Activity 3.2.3a.

You may be called upon to lecture in your College of Nursing/ Midwifery. Think what factors you need to consider when preparing for this.

First you might need to ask if this is the most appropriate format for teaching the particular topic. You should remember that lectures are often used to give information which is readily available in textbooks or in distance learning packages, in which case the student may be more fruitfully occupied seeking the information from this source. If students are directed towards the primary source initially, then they can seek the assistance of the teacher to check understanding, or the implications for practice.

If lecturing is not the mode of choice, or the most appropriate format, you need to select a different approach. Let us assume that a 'lecture' *is* the most appropriate method.

Activity 3.2.3b.

List the factors you need to consider in order to plan your session to
ensure maximum benefit for the students.

Your list may look something like this:
   type of course
   previous experience of students
   educational background of students
   size of class
   where the session will be held
   scope of content to be taught
   strategies for maintaining students' attention
   strategies for aiding retention of information
   teacher/student relationship.
Having prepared your list, let us now take identified considerations and
explore them in more depth.

Activity 3.2.3c.

Why is it important to know about the type of course?

1.   This gives you the information you need in order to plan your
     session at an appropriate level. For example, as a teacher-prac-
     titioner working in the Accident and Emergency Department you
     may be asked to talk about triage. The level of information you
     would plan to teach would vary considerably between that which
     you would share with students about to enter the Department for
     clinical experience and qualified staff undertaking a National
     Board Accident and Emergency Nursing Course. You will be able to
     think of examples which are relevant to your own area of practice.

2.   Once you have established the level it enables you to collect appro-
     priate data/references/research, etc.

3. You can impart information about the level at which you are teaching into your introduction indicating an interest in the group.

Activity 3.2.3d.

What about the students' previous experience? How will knowing this help you?

---

1. This allows you to make certain assumptions about where the student is at, in terms of their professional development. Remember, though, that this is an assumption. You cannot be sure that every qualified nurse, say, has had experience with dying patients, or at resuscitation.

2. You can relate your session to existing knowledge and so build on this. This is an extremely important principle in teaching: if you assume knowledge that is not there, learning will fail to occur; if you pitch your teaching at to low a level, you run the risk of appearing to patronise the learners.

3. You have an idea of what they already know and this will help you to plan your approach to the topic and determine the level of information more appropriately.

Activity 3.2.3e.

Why is it important to know the educational background of the students?

You need to know whether the students are:
graduates
diplomates
1st or 2nd level practitioners
students on pre-registration courses.

You need to know:
    their range of academic qualifications
    whether they have undertaken post-registration courses.
Knowing this will help you select appropriate language and determine the
amount of explanation that is required.

Activity 3.2.3f.

Why is it important to know the size of the class?

This knowledge will help you with your planning in terms of preparing:
    handouts
    the sort of learning activities you may wish to include
    the visual aids you can use
    seating arrangements
Remember that small groups are often better in comfortable chairs
arranged in a semi-circle, or failing that, desks and chairs in a similar
arrangement.
    In essence, it helps you to prepare yourself and take into account things
like:
    pitching your voice so that everyone can hear
    how you present yourself so that everyone can see
    how you maintain eye contact with all members of a large group
    how you will integrate questions into the session.
You will also need to know so that when you enter the teaching room you
are neither overawed by the number nor disappointed.

Activity 3.2.3g.

Think about what you need to know about the physical setting for
your session and draw up a list.

Your list will probably look something like this:
venue
desks/chairs/tables
chalkboard/whiteboard—chalk/pens
overhead projector/pens
flip chart/pens
television/video/camera
slide projector
simulation mannequin
display boards
Obviously the equipment you require will depend on what you intend to do.

Activity 3.2.3h.

Take time out and make an appointment to visit your College of Nursing/Midwifery to meet the audio-visual aids technician. Whilst you're with her, ask about the equipment and how to use it— properly. You will find this useful and it will help you when using learning aids in your session.

It may be pertinent, since we have mentioned learning aids, to offer a few tips on their preparation and how you can use them effectively to help students retain information.

Audio-visual aids to learning

Why use audio-visual resources?
Audio-visual aids play an important role in education both as a tool for learning and an avenue for experience.

Visual aids and technology have several functions. They:
(a) enhance clarity of communication
(b) provide diversity in teaching methods
(c) aid retention
(d) give impact
(e) provide experiences not normally available
(f) simulate real life situations
(g) permit practice and so give confidence
(h) use a range of senses
(i) increase and sustain attention

(j)   provide realism
(k)   increase the meaningfulness of abstract concepts.

Principles underlying the successful use of recourses
Having said that, if audio-visual resources are to optimise learning, then they must be:
(a)   of good quality
(b)   relevant
(c)   flexible
(d)   simple
(e)   available, transportable and storable
(f)   cheap to produce, buy, loan or hire
(g)   well-planned
(h)   within the limits of the law (e.g. not infringe copyright law)
(i)   colourful or eye-catching
(j)   of a suitable size

Types of learning aids available
1.   Field trips

2.   Graphic aids
     —   flip charts
     —   cards
     —   diagrams
     —   cartoons
     —   overhead transparencies
     —   flannel boards
     —   magnetic boards
     —   posters
     —   chalk boards

3.   Education exhibits
     —   demonstrations
     —   exhibitions
     —   specimens

4.   Still pictures
     —   photographs
     —   plans
     —   slides
     —   pictures

5.   Programmed learning
     —   books
     —   cards
     —   games

6. Radio

7. Recordings
   — home-made
   — bought or hired

8. Television
   — VCR equipment
   — TV broadcasts

9. Films

10. Working models

11. 'The real thing'
    — patients
    — equipment

12. Computers

Sources of visual aid materials

1. College of Nursing/Midwifery: usually have
   — models
   — charts
   — films
   — materials to make aids
   — books
   — film strips
   — tape recorders
   — overhead projectors
   — boards (chalk and white)
   — computers

2. Institutions, voluntary organisations and commercial firms, such as drug or appliance manufacturers, organisations such as the Health Education Authority or the British Heart Foundation, can often supply free items such as:

   — posters
   — slides
   — tapes
   — models
   — books
   — handouts
   — diagrams

3.   Film hire companies: Because of the cost of hire (up to £100 a day) you would be advised to approach the College of Nursing/Midwifery.

No doubt you will be able to think of other possible resources but this should have given you some information about the scope of learning aids. When you set about creating learning aids to enhance your teaching, your College of Nursing or Midwifery will probably be only too pleased to help and advise.

Before you prepare your learning aids, you need to organise the content of your session so that you can determine exactly what you need and where in your session you will use them for maximum impact. You also need to consider the sequencing of your session and the depth and diversity of information you will include.

Identifying what to teach

Activity 3.2.3i.

In order to help you do this we will take a hypothetical situation.

You are approached by your College of Nursing/Midwifery to undertake a session. (You need here to decide what it is you are going to teach—perhaps you would wish to use a topic you selected for the activities undertaken in chapter 1)

Now choose *one* of the following alternatives.

This session is for a group of pre-registration students, nine months into their programme. The placement in your area will be their second placement, the first having been undertaken in the community.

or

The session is to be undertaken for a group of post-registration students undertaking a National Board course. They are all qualified practitioners with at least six months' post-qualifying experience

or

if you yourself are undertaking a Project 2000 course, imagine you are to prepare a session for a group of school leavers who have expressed an interest in nursing.

Before you start to plan your session refer to your brief outline of a teaching plan. Using this plan as a guide, you need to consider carefully what it is you intend to include in your session. This is not as easy as it sounds, and it may take you some time to get your ideas together. You may decide to put your information on paper in the form of a spider graph or rough notes—choose the method which suits you best. Put everything you can think of onto your paper. Next you need to visit your college library and start to locate a range of appropriate, up-to-date literature. If you ask the librarian, s/he will probably help and may do a literature search for you.

Start off by thinking of those whom you are going to teach as knowing absolutely nothing; once you have all the information you require about the group, you can begin to delete information that is inappropriate to their needs.

To help you with your session you need to remember that to be effective your session must include things the student

must learn

should learn

could learn

If your student only learns the information she *could/should* learn without what she *must* learn, then your session is not effective. For example, imagine that for your birthday you received an expensively wrapped gift, only to discover on opening it that it was an empty box. Alternatively suppose someone close to you gave you expensive perfume/aftershave in an unattractive package. Neither of these two alternatives would be satisfactory as a present. If, however, you received a beautifully wrapped gift and upon opening you discover expensive perfume, then you would be happy.

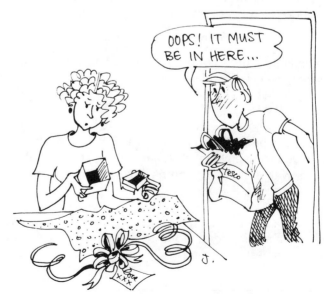

This analogy is included to show that if you prepare a session and you do not add some 'wrapping and packaging' to make it interesting, then it is potentially very dry and unmotivating and the effectiveness of the learning is lessened. On the other hand, if the session is well-packaged but does not actually achieve what you set out to achieve, then it has the same result.

Activity 3.2.3j.

If you have just 15 minutes to teach the important points of your chosen teaching topic, what would those points be?

What would you add to this list if you had 90 minutes?

What about if the college asked you to do a series of sessions on the same subject over three half-days?

How different are your lists?

This activity should have helped you to formulate what you

> *must*
> *should*
> *could* teach

There are some other factors which you need to consider when planning your session:

Is your knowledge adequate?
Do you need to expand/update your knowledge?
What is the most up-to-date research on the topic?
Do you have the references for it?
Who do you know, who is an expert, from whom you can seek advice?
How best can you make your point? (Start listening to other people teaching to glean ideas and tips.)
How will you know what the students have learned?
What strategies can you employ if someone asks you an awkward question?

Planning your session will take a good deal of time, but like all events which are planned carefully and with precision, the likelihood of problems is minimised—minimised you will notice, NOT eradicated. In teaching there is always the possibility of an unanticipated question or response, but that is what makes teaching exciting. If you have planned carefully, extended your own knowledge and prepared your teaching notes, then you are on firm ground and can direct the session the way you want it to go. Alternatively, you can, if you feel confident enough, let the session go the way the students want it to go, which may be in a completely different direction. If you do this, though, remember that the direction still has to be relevant to meeting the students' expected learning outcomes.

Some other considerations

Clearly you will want to engage the students in interaction, so try writing your questions out in your teaching notes so that you do not have to try and formulate questions when you are under stress. Questioning techniques require a great deal of practice if you are consistently to frame your questions so that they bring forth the answers you want.

If it is your intention to draw a flowchart or diagram using the chalk/white board or flip chart, then you would be well advised to practise drawing the complete diagram on paper the same shape as the board you are using, then you can see where you need to place your first markings and subsequent additions without running out of board. The way in which you introduce yourself and the session will set the tone. Try to create an atmosphere of anticipation and excitement. If you are enthusiastic about the topic, then this will rub off on your students.

Each teacher has his/her own style and you are now starting to develop yours.

Walters and Marks (1981) suggest that there are three kinds of lecture:

The ideal . . . attendance is voluntary with the participants being there because they want to be which indicates commitment. The values and beliefs of both lecturer and participant are shared.

The classical . . . attendance is compulsory and the session is very specific in its subject matter.

The experimental . . . used prior to activities and intended to give the participants information about the issues in question.

Activity 3.2.3k

How is teaching approached in your College of Nursing/Midwifery?

Why not visit and see if you can attend some of the sessions.

Compare these with those you remember from your student days.

How have they changed?

Whatever methods you employ in your teaching there will be occasions when you are required to give explanations; it is also very difficult to imagine any teaching/learning situation without questions.

Perhaps this is an appropriate time to stop and consider both.

Explaining

Brown and Armstrong (1984) define explaining as 'an attempt to provide understanding of a problem to others' and give three types of explanation:

1. interpretive: answers 'what' questions

2. descriptive: answers 'how' questions

3. reason-giving: answers 'why' questions

The following sequence for planning is adapted from Brown (1978) in Quinn (1988).
(a)   You need to decide exactly what is to be explained.
(b)   Identify those concepts which may not be obvious and which may influence understanding, for example, in explaining how oxygen gets from the air to the tissues, you would identify the concept of diffusion of gases and gaseous exchange.
(c)   Highlight the key points.
(d)   Write a simple statement for each key point.
(e)   Summarise the key points.
(f)   Prepare the introduction. The rationale for this is that once you have formulated the explanation you are in a position to engender interest.

Questioning

Brown and Edmundsen (1984) define this as 'any statement intended to evoke a verbal response'.

Activity 3.2.3I.

What do you consider to be the purpose of questions in teaching?

Check your ideas against Quinn's (1988) below.

'Purposes of educational questioning
These can be grouped under four main headings:

1. Social purposes:
    to promote active involvement of the learners during a lesson;
    to encourage closer relationships between teachers and learners;
    to elicit any special interests or experience from the learners, for
    example 'Has anyone nursed a patient with this condition?'

2. Motivational purposes:
    to develop the learners' interest and motivation, for example,
    'How do you think that this problem might be overcome?'
    to focus attention upon an aspect of the lecture;
    to provide a change of stimulus during a lecture.

3. Cognitive purposes:
    to encourage the learners to think at varying levels of complexity,
    and in a logical, analytical way.

4. Assessment purposes:
    to assess the previous knowledge or skill of a learner;
    to assess the learner's ability to use the higher levels of cognitive
    functioning such as synthesis, analysis and evaluation;
    to provide the teacher with feedback on the learning taking place
    during the course of a lecture.'

So, how can you make your questioning more effective? In essence, good
questions should

—   be short,

—   be stated in language that the student understands

—   be appropriate to the level of the student

—   be unambiguous

—   seek a response to only one point

—   be open-ended, that is, requiring more than a yes/no answer.

Activity 3.2.3m.

Apply the above criteria to some questions you formulate and then
try them out on either colleagues or students and note the response.

The important point to consider is whether your questions draw forth the response you required, that is, did they meet your purpose?

Teaching Small Groups of Students

There are different types of small teaching groups in which you may be involved and a variety of techniques you may wish to employ.

Tutorial Groups

Tutorial groups could be an encounter with one or more students and you. The purpose of the group will determine how the group is organised. For example, the group may wish to explore various strategies for attempting an assignment, in which case each group member may present a different approach.

Seminar

The seminar is mainly concerned with academic matters, usually involving the presentation of a paper or essay by a student followed by group discussion. Although this type of session is mainly focused on the students, the teacher needs to have a sound grasp of the material being presented and an ability to lead the group in analysing and evaluating this.

Activity 3.2.3n.

Can you think of any situations in the clinical area when you may wish to use either a tutorial or a seminar?

For example, you could use a tutorial to help students to formulate care plans, write reports, prepare case conferences or as part of demonstrating a skill.

A seminar could be used, possibly over a lunch time with the care-team, to explore one problematic aspect of a client's care, for example, the management of intractable pain.

Discussion groups

Discussion groups can be either controlled or free. The leadership in controlled groups is assumed by the teacher, in order to explain any difficulties the students may have related to subject matter. Free discussion groups are student-led, this may increase students' motivation by giving them responsibility for their own learning.

Problem-solving groups
The main purpose of this type of group is to encourage critical thinking. A common strategy is to present a case study of a patient/client. The group then sets out to explore that person's problems and the ways in which they might be tackled. Other techniques such as brainstorming might be used within the group. You may like to find out from your College of Nursing or Midwifery what other types of group-encounter are being used. You will need to speak to several members of the teaching staff, since each one may have his or her favourite approach and it will be of benefit to you to find out about as many as you can.

Brainstorming
An intensive discussion in which spontaneous suggestions as solutions to a problem are accepted uncritically. The suggestions are written down without any attempt to order or evaluate them. After all the suggestions have been made, the group uses them to reach a consensus about the best solution to the problem. This method can lead to some imaginative approaches and the formulation of several options.

Buzz groups
Two to six group members are asked to discuss issues or problems for a short period of time within a lesson. A reporter from each group then presents their findings to the whole. This method can be useful in encouraging students who are shy or reticent, encouraging group cohesion, getting the group motivated, focusing their attention on pertinent issues and in encouraging the development of interpersonal skills or discussion techniques.

Case discussion
Where real or simulated problems related to individual patients/clients are analysed in detail, with the participating care-team members contributing their own solutions or proposals and decisions. This method is valuable in facilitating an understanding of interrelationships within the multidisciplinary team.

Projects
A project usually consists of an exercise submitted on paper in the form of an essay, backed up with audio-visual resources, which is frequently accompanied by a verbal synopsis of the findings. It can be undertaken singly or in a group. Project work uses information-seeking skills, and an ability to organise, apply and present information in a relevant format.

Experiential learning methods

Earlier in this chapter an initial identification of the characteristics of experiential learning was undertaken.

Activity 3.2.3n.

Without referring to this list can you remember them?

Using this list as a foundation, you need to reflect on what using experiential learning methods in the clinical areas means to you as a practitioner-teacher. In the concluding chapter of this book you will have the opportunity to explore the possible ways of introducing experiential learning methods into your clinical area in relation to teaching models/frameworks for nursing and midwifery practice. The emphasis of this method is on action, i.e. the student learns through the processes of the activity as opposed to the more traditional forms of learning, where the student is a passive recipient. The role of the teacher is not to dispense knowledge (Gray 1986) but rather to help the student to make sense of his or her experience.

Students can learn *through* experience or they can learn *from* experience.

Activity 3.2.3o.

Can you think of any instances in which you have learned through experience and also in which you have learned from experience?

Here are a couple of examples to start you off.

Learning *through* experience: Think of an occasion when you have been a patient, perhaps sitting in the Out-patient or Accidents and Emergency Department. Has this affected the way in which you now deliver care?

Learning *from* experience: Look back, for a moment, to the time when you first became a staff-nurse or first had responsibility for organising the nursing/midwifery team in your area. How has what you learned from that experience affected the way in which you now relate to other staff members?

This chapter is designed as a resource to help you when you plan your teaching. We hope that you will refer to it often when deciding, first of all, the overall approach which you will take, and then the methods you will employ within the approach. Assessing the needs of the learners and planning teaching to meet those needs, using effective strategies, is crucial to success in both teaching and learning.

GLOSSARY

Gaming: closely related to role play and simulation but differs in that it usually has a set of precise rules and is competitive in nature. Unlike role play and simulation, gaming does not have a scenario, participants behave as themselves. Educational games are extensions of recreational games.

Operant conditioning: differs from classical conditioning in that the learned behaviour is instrumental in controlling the experiencing organism's environment.

Psychomotor skills: involve both intellectual skills and motor skills in order to be able to execute the procedure.

Role play: utilises acting and imagination to give insight into the student's own behaviour values/beliefs, by creating a scenario in which the student 'acts out' a situation.

Simulation: closely associated with role play, but essentially the student remains 'herself' throughout the situation, responding in the way she sees as appropriate.

REFERENCES

Bandura A (1977) *Social Learning Theory*. Englewood Cliffs, NJ: Prentice Hall.
Beard R, Bligh D and Harding A (1978) *Research into Teaching Methods in Higher Education* (4th edn). Surrey: Society for Research into Higher Education.
Benner P (1984) *From Novice to Expert*. California: Addison Wesley.
Bevis E (1982) *Curriculum Building in Nursing*. St Louis: Mosby.
Bligh D (1972) *What's the Use of Lectures?* London: Penguin.
Bloom B (1964) *A Handbook of Educational Objectives—The Cognitive Domain*. New York: McKay.
Brown G (1978) *Lecturing and Explaining*, cited in Quinn (1988). London: Methuen.
Brown G and Armstrong S (1984) Explaining and Explanation. In *Classroom Teaching Skills*, E Wragg (Ed). London: Croom Helm.
Brown G and Edmundson P (1984) Asking Questions. In *Classroom Teaching Skills*, E Wragg (Ed). London: Croom Helm.

Burnard P (1990) *Learning Human Skills: An Experimental Guide for Nurses* (2nd edn). Oxford: Heinemann.

Burrel T (1988) *Curriculum Design and Development*. London: Prentice Hall.

Davies I K (1976) *Objectives in Curriculum Design*. London: McGraw Hill.

Fitts P and Posner M (1967) *Human Performance*. Englewood Cliffs, NJ: Prentice Hall.

Fretwell J E (1980) An Enquiry into the Ward Learning Envinronment. *Nursing Times*, **76**(16), 69–75.

Gagne R (1983) *The Conditions of Learning and Theory of Instruction* (4th edn). New York: Holt Rinehart and Winston.

Gibson (1980) A Critique of the Objectives Model in Curriculum Design. *Journal of Advanced Nursing*, **5**(2), 161–7.

Gott M (1983) *Preparation of the Student for Learning in the Clinical Setting*. London: Royal College of Nursing.

Gott M (1984) *Learning Nursing*. London: Royal College of Nursing.

Gray H (1986) Experiential Learning with Adults, Self and Society. *European Journal of Humanistic Psychology*, **4**(6), 282–286.

Jarvis P (1988) *Adult and Continuing Education: Theory and Practice*. London: Routledge and Kegan Paul.

Knowles M (1970) *The Modern Practice of Adult Education Androgogy v Pedagogy*. Chicago: Follet.

Knowles M (1973) *The Adult Learner. A neglected species*. Houston: Gulf Publishing.

Knowles M (1984) *Andragogy in Action*. San Francisco: Jossey Barr.

Krathwohl D (1968) *A Handbook of Educational Objectives: The Affective Domain*. New York: McKay.

Marson S N (1982) Ward Sister, Teacher or Facilitator? An investigation into behavioural characteristics of effective ward teachers. *Journal of Advanced Nursing*, **7**, 347–357.

Ogier M E (1982) *An Ideal Sister?* London: Royal College of Nursing.

Ogier M E (1986) An Ideal Sister—Seven years on. Occasional Paper. *Nursing Times*, **82**(2), 54–57.

Ogier M E and Barnett (1986) Sister Staff Nurse and the Nurse Learner. *Nurse Education Today*, **6**, 16–22.

Orton H D (1981) Ward Learning Climate and Student Nurse Response. Occasional Paper. *Nursing Times*, **77**(23), 65–68.

Quinn F M (1988) *The Principles and Practice of Nurse Education* (2nd edn). London: Croom Helm.

Rogers C (1969) *Freedom to Learn*. Ohio: Merrill.

Rogers C (1983) *Freedom to Learn for the 80's*. Ohio: Merrill.

Sheahan J (1978) Ward Sister: Manager, Nurse or Teacher? *Nursing Mirror*, **135**, 18–21.

Simpson E (1966) *Classification of Educational Objectives: The Psychomotor Domain*. University of Illinois.

Skinner B F (1968) *The Technology of Teaching*. New York: Appleton-Century-Croft.

Steinaker N and Bell (1979) *The Experiential Taxonomy: A New Approach to Teaching and Learning*. London: Academic Press.

UKCC (1984) *Code of Professional Conduct for Nurse, Midwife and Health Visitor.* London: UKCC

UKCC (1986) *Project 2000: A New Preparation for Practice.* London: UKCC.

UKCC (1990) *The Report of the Post Registration Education and Practice Project.* London: UKCC.

Walters G and Marks S (1981) *Experiential Learning and Change: Theory, Development and Practice.* Chichester: Wiley.

Wong J (1979) The Inability to Transfer. Classroom learning to clinical nursing practice: a learning problem and its remedial plan. *Journal of Advanced Nurses,* **4**, 161–168.

FURTHER READING

Hinchliff S M (Ed) (1986) *Teaching Clinical Nursing* (2nd edn). Edinburgh: Churchill Livingstone. This comprehensive book explores the process of clinical nursing and the role of the teacher in clinical areas including psychiatry and paediatrics. It is a valuable resource for you to use.

Kenworthy N and Nicklin P (1989) *Teaching and Assessing in Nursing Practice: An experiential approach.* London: Scutari Press. This book is well worth reading. It gives an introduction to the experiential taxonomy and how it can be applied to nurse education by exploring the principles of teaching and learning, methods of assessing, developments in nurse education and the nature and purpose of evaluation. As Eve Bendall wrote in her foreword to this book 'Neil Kenworthy and Peter Nicklin belong to the generation of Directors of Nurse Education in whose hands will lie the greatest transition ever envisaged for nurse training'.

Ogier M E (1989) *Working and Learning: The learning environment in clinical nursing.* London: Scutari Press. A very useful book for you to dip into and to help you with your teaching in clinical areas. It explores such issues as learning in the clinical area, creating a learning environment, and puts forward some ideas for teaching in the clinical area. The book also contains a section containing exercises for the reader and comprehensive suggestions for further reading.

Selecting books

Books are very personal to the reader, and as such it would be worth your while visiting your college library and browsing through the shelves. The listed suggestions are by no means the only books on the shelves relating to the subject of teaching and learning, but are the ones which the author finds particularly interesting.

Within your library there are probably a number of journals which, up to now, you may not have considered to be relevant to your practice. Try to get into the habit of going to the library and scanning the most recent copies. In particular, look out for *Nurse Education Today.*

Chapter 4

The Process of Teaching and Learning

Whatever your areas of practice, your teaching expertise or the course/ position your 'student' is on or in, there are many factors which will impinge on the effectiveness of your teaching. This chapter endeavours to look at some of these aspects and how you might recognise and manage them in order to improve your teaching.

When you are teaching, you will need to assess your students' language ability, their cultural background, their individual differences and their academic ability, along with the level of course they are studying, where appropriate. The potential combinations of these factors are complex and pose a challenge to the teacher in adapting her teaching to meet the learners' needs.

The consequences of ignoring them are that the student may feel alienated from the teacher and the student's full potential will not be developed. This will not happen if the teacher recognises that teaching is an interactive process which requires sensitivity to all the student's needs. Remember, your student may be anyone from a patient/client to a fellow professional requiring your expertise in a particular area, and their age may range from toddler to ninety.

SOCIOLOGICAL FACTORS INFLUENCING TEACHING

Language

The study of language is known as philology and languages fall into three main groups: Indo-European, Chinese and Semitic. Everyone has their own idiolect within these groups, that is, a combination of accent and **dialect.**

Dialect refers to a collection of linguistic items which can be identified regionally and by social class. For example, the use of double negatives is a working-class tendency. Difference in dialects is not linguistic however, but has social class overtones.

Most of us would recognise a different **accent** and be able to identify its origin quite easily. Some accents tend to be thought of as more socially acceptable than others, and some are perceived as being associated with higher levels of intelligence or ability. For example, a received pronunciation accent (the sort of accent commonly heard in television newscasters) is generally regarded as socially acceptable and perceived by many as being a measure of intelligence and social class.

Basil Bernstein (1960, 1962), an American sociologist, suggests causal links between social class, family structure, socialisation and education. He defines two main linguistic codes and relates them to these concepts.

Bernstein argues that working-class people use a restricted language code (that is, they use a limited vocabulary with curtailed speech constructions) and this results in a lack of cognitive meaning in their speech. This is thought to have an effect on how the person can understand and relate to the outside world. People who have restricted language codes tend to find themselves at a disadvantage in an educational setting, since most teachers used an elaborated language code.

Bernstein defined this elaborated language code, which is attributed to the middle and upper classes, as the opposite of a restricted code, involving use of an extensive vocabulary and a richer range of speech forms.

Bernstein's work draws on a modified version of work by Whorf (1956), who developed the theory that a society is ordered in a particular way because of the structure of its language. That is to say, the world is perceived through the filter of language.

Activity 4.1.

Try to remember what it was like when you first started nursing or midwifery, before you acquired a grasp of professional language, e.g. you may have known what it was like for someone to have a stroke, but did not know what a cerebro-vascular accident was. Reflect on how lost you often felt.

You may remember that you first thought of a stroke as a kind of paralysis and had no idea of what caused it. The purpose of this activity is to ensure that you remember to explain clearly to your students any term you think they may not know.

Activity 4.2.

Reflect on different accents that you hear in the UK, and write down those that you find unpleasant or unacceptable. Why do you feel like this?

You need not show your answer to anyone and you should try to be quite honest.

It is important that you are aware that you may unfairly attribute certain qualities to your students because of their accents. Becoming more aware of this potential tendency should help you to be more objective in your relationships.

The teacher also needs to consider language and meaning. Meanings involve shared understandings. Wittgenstein (1953), a philosopher, pointed out that we cannot have a private language; all languages carry meanings and have social implications and connotations which are constantly reinforced by communication. Meanings are rooted in social, economic and historical contexts and are socially structured; for example, the word 'wealth' may mean something entirely different to the owner of an Elizabethan mansion, compared with an unemployed steel worker.

It is important to realise that there is no research to prove that there is a relationship between language and cognitive ability; however, it is clear that you cannot understand something if you do not have the language for it. A word of caution is needed here for the teacher, in that your student may have a different word (language) for what you are trying to describe. In other words, you may both be familiar with the matter under discussion, but be unable to communciate because of a difference in language. An interesting point to consider is Labon's (1970) view that we are all multi-dialectic or multi-stylistic, and that people intuitively adapt to suit the social situation. An example of this is when people adopt a 'telephone' voice. When people do not adapt socially, it is probably because they are identifying with a different social group within the situation, e.g. children in hospital may relate to their peer group linguistically, rather then to the nurse or doctor.

The language we use within the health care profession is in elaborated code. Our professional language also uses standard English. These factors are important when trying to teach people who may not have this language facility, e.g. some patients or clients. Remember, then, to assess your student properly before you start teaching, in order that you avoid a speech style that either is 'above their heads' or 'talks down to them'. Either approach would be quite unacceptable and inconducive to learning.

Culture

Any student group will link into a **culture** or **sub-culture** of one type or another. For example, taking patients or clients as a group, they tend to identify with one another in terms of common problems and we encourage this by introducing them to self-help groups. The teacher needs to understand the accepted values, attitude and behaviour of the culture or sub-culture in order to establish a rapport with the student. Mead (1934) says that we all start off by learning roles from our parents then complete our socialisation by internalising (that is, accepting as our own) the norms and values of other membership groups, both at the cultural and sub-cultural level. We also tend to become labelled by others according to the cultures and sub-cultures we ourselves operate in.

The influences brought to bear culturally on students are of enormous consequence, since they may be of far greater importance to the student than those imparted by the teacher. For example, their relationship to their **peer group** is very important to adolescents and they would often rather please their peers than their family or teachers. Many students in the Health Service are adolescents, and therefore much of what the teacher tries to achieve will be of no consequence if it is not accepted by the peer group.

For instance, if you had a group of students with whom to discuss Health Promotion, you would have to estimate the influence of their peer group. Suppose your session was to be on smoking, it would be easier to demonstrate the ill-effects of smoking to a group where the peer group does not smoke, and where their original socialisation to non-smoking behaviour was because their parents did not smoke. It would obviously be considerably harder to convince a group of the ill-effects of smoking if their parents had always smoked and members of their peer group did.

The strongest influence with children at the pre-adolescent stage is parental. The most influential factor for adults is largely related to self, having evolved over the years from other influences which have been modified, adjusted and replaced. Remember, though, that the peer group still exerts some influence over decision-making.

In theory, the teacher should find it easier to teach adults, since negotiation and bargaining with the student is on a one-to-one, face-to-face level.

Activity 4.3.

Think of five issues related to health where you would need to consider the influence of the student's peer group. In completing the activity consider the consequences of the individual conforming.

For example, drug abusers who are admitted to hospital may present the practitioner-teacher with a dilemma. She must ignore how she feels about drug abuse in order to discuss the individual's problems with them. For their part, the practitioner-teacher is asking that the drug abuser abandon the values, behaviour patterns of their own sub-cultural peer group.

Certain cultures produce deviant (that is unacceptably aberrant) behaviour simply because they do not fit in with the cultural norms of society as a whole. For example, criminal behaviour is determined by the society in which you live; what is criminal behaviour in our society may not be regarded as such in another. In the Health Service, the practitioner may be faced with deviant behaviour and must be non-judgemental in order to generate an effective learning situation.

Loyalty to peers is extremely important in cultural sub-groups, since neglect of this causes rejection by other group members. However, students are generally prepared to negotiate with their teacher to make for a more comfortable working environment. A student who is good at negotiating may be more likely to succeed. For example, if a student is unable to negotiate extra time to complete an assignment, he or she may fail even though having legitimate reasons for an extended submission date.

The influence of negotiating skills can be extended; good negotiators seem to be able to do no wrong, often termed the 'halo effect', whereas poor negotiators seem to do everything wrong—the so-called 'horns effect'.

The teacher also needs to negotiate the context of the situation in which he or she is teaching. For example, a certain amount of noise may be acceptable and beyond that conflict may exist. It is unlikely that practitioner-teachers will face noise problems, although interruptions may disrupt teaching sessions and negotiation may be appropriate here.

Students who do not conform to their teacher's expectations do not always do well, falling into the trap of not achieving highly because they are not expected to. Merton (1957) described this situation as the self-fulfilling prophecy. This describes the situation when the teacher constantly tells a student that she is performing poorly. The student comes to believe in this 'prophecy' and this belief affects her performance adversely. The prophecy is thus fulfilled by the student.

The implication of this for the practitioner-teacher is that positive reinforcement (i.e. praise) should be used to ensure the continuance of effective learning, and all criticism should be clear, constructive and non-personal.

It may be an expectation, on the part of the teacher, that their authority/ experience is in no way questioned. The practitioner-teacher in health care will need to guard against seeing this as an example of students being 'difficult', since a questioning attitude is one which should be actively encouraged today in nursing and midwifery education. It also goes without saying that if we are to respect clients' and patients' views, then we must be prepared to be challenged and respond professionally.

Understanding

In any teaching situation the practitioner as a teacher should bear in mind the range of socio-linguistic and socio-cultural factors mentioned above, since they may be important in determining student success.

As an example, assume you are working in a ward caring for elderly clients, and you need to teach a lady how to manage a venous leg ulcer. The lady has scant knowledge of things medical and it would therefore be of little use to explain care in purely professional terms. Culturally, this person also believes that she should leave her caring to the professionals. Therefore, in order to gain her co-operation in planning her care, you will need to avoid terms that make her think you want her to do your job for you!

In contrast, take a social worker in her late 30s who is your client. Obviously with this person it would be entirely appropriate to use professional language as long as you remember that she may have difficulties with some specific terms. Should this be the case, you will need to observe for signs of uncertainty, since some people are unwilling to admit that they do not understand if someone appears to think that they should. In this particular situation, cultural problems are unlikely.

In further contrast, take your immediate senior manager and think of one aspect of your role which you understand very well and on which your superior is seeking clarifiction. Socio-linguistically you can use professional language but you will need to take care to achieve a balance between assuming what is already known and the gaps that need filling in or elaborating on. It is potentially difficult, in this situation, to avoid stating what may already be obvious and losing your student's interest! Socio-culturally, you, as the teacher, may feel in an inferior position; traditionally the teacher occupies a superior position; however, in adult learning situations the position of teacher and taught tend to be equal. If you do not pay attention to these factors, you will find that your student switches off, does not respect your abilities as a teacher and may concentrate less on what you have to say in the future.

This situation is particularly dangerous where issues of health and safety are at risk, for example, where a patient needs to understand the possible side-effects of a drug she is taking, or a relative needs to be taught safe lifting techniques. It is therefore inappropriate for any teacher to fail to give credence to factors of language and culture.

PSYCHOLOGICAL INFLUENCES ON NATURE V NURTURE

Learning is a complex activity and is different from maturation (i.e. the process of growth and development). Learning occurs as a result of a combination of factors related to memory, perception and motivation. The Nature v Nurture debate originated in philosophy and is taken up in psychology under the heading of genetic and environmental influences on learning. Unquestionably people vary in intellectual ability, but how much of this is due to the genes they inherit or the environment in which they are brought up? Most experts agree that at least some aspects of intelligence are inherited (Thomas and Chess 1977), the debate focuses on how much is hereditary and how much is due to environmental influences. Readers should consult a psychology text such as Atkinson et al (1990) for a full analysis of the debate.

Individual Differences

Many differences have already been noted. Individuals who conform to society's norms generally receive more positive responses from teachers. Temperament is an individual difference relevant to the teacher. Ill-tempered individuals tend not to bring out the best response in teachers. The practitioner-teacher will have to control her own response to this type of behaviour, in order to convey the necessary information and ensure that it is understood.

Given that environmental influences are very important with regard to intelligence, the teacher can obviously facilitate these with the correct techniques. For example, in trying to teach a particular concept to a client, there are several factors to consider. Bruner (1974) defined these as follows:

1. *Defining the task*:   the teacher should attempt to define this very clearly. That is, the student must know what is to be taught and how it is to be taught.

2. *The nature of the learning situation*:   the type of situation and its context affects how soon or how well the concept is learned.

3. *The nature of validation*:   that is, is what you are planning to teach a valid representation of the concept? A skill is easier to learn if steps can be traced, and if the student can move from the known to the unknown in a step-wise fashion.

4. *The consequences of specific categorisations*:   there is a cost to categorising wrongly, that is, the concept will not be learned accurately. For example, if a technique has not been categorised as an aseptic technique and it should have been, then that technique will have been learned ineffectively.

5. *The nature of imposed restrictions*:   e.g. pressure of time, the teacher needs to attend to any restrictions and ensure that the student is not disadvantaged.

Deductive and inductive learning

People can learn inductively by studying theory and problem-solving, or deductively, by learning from experience. The teacher-practitioner can aid this process by ensuring that the student is taught the correct theory and given as much experience in the related subject as possible.

When planning to teach a concept to any student, the teacher-practitioner must consider the following aspects:

1. First identify the concepts and decide which order they should be taught in. For example, the student first needs a concept of infection before the concept of cross-infection can be dealt with.

2. Decide which concepts should be taught deductively and which should be taught inductively. For example, the concept of infection could be taught inductively whilst cross-infection could be taught inductively and deductively.

3. It may be essential that the student actually experiences the concept, and so when teaching cross-infection, **Agar plates** may be obtained from the laboratory and you could demonstrate how organisms can be transferred by hands or uniform. The teacher can teach deductively by showing the student rules or examples and then suggest the student creates her own definition and relates this to other concepts.

4. You will also need to assess whether your student thinks in concrete terms and is likely to have difficulty with abstract concepts. In this case you will need to think of some concrete examples to represent the abstract concept.

Activity 4.4.

Think of a topic you might have to teach, e.g. how to communicate effectively with relatives. How might this be demonstrated to a student? What strategies would you use to teach this concept, i.e. inductive, deductive or both? How could you evaluate what the student had learned? What would you do if the student had not learned?

If you feel that you managed this piece of teaching effectively, give yourself a pat on the back. If it did not work out quite as well as you hoped, spend some time reflecting on why this was so and planning how you could improve on your performance the next time you teach it.

Teaching a Skill

Although this topic is also covered in chapter 3 on planning teaching, we are including here aspects relevant to the process of teaching.

When teaching a skill you will first need to analyse the stages, demonstrate them and get your student to carry out the skill under your supervision.

Skills involve both cognitive (thinking) and motor (dexterity) aspects. The practitioner-teacher will need to ensure that the student does not become too tired or bored when learning a skill and must be aware of any drugs which may affect the student's performance. This is particularly pertinent when the person being taught is a patient or client. If the student' performance is reduced, then the teacher should endeavour to make the subject more interesting and go at a pace which is appropriate for the student.

Activity 4.5.

Imagine you are to teach someone how to give an intramuscular injection. Break down the skill into component parts to represent the steps of the total skill. Remember to state stages that appear obvious, like remove the syringe from its wrapper, without contaminating the syringe.

continued on next page

continued ───

> Consider how you might teach the activity in an interesting way.
> Remember not to give too much information, you are purely teaching
> the skill not including concepts such as asepsis.

Were you surprised at the number of steps involved? Ineffective teaching occurs when too many steps are taught together or when steps are omitted. Clearly you do not have infinite time at your disposal when teaching a skill in the clinical area, but nevertheless, you should take a few moments to reflect on the skill, the steps involved and the needs of the person to whom you are to teach it.

Attributes necessary for sport and manual skills can all be related to the sort of motor skills that are met in clinical practice and are as follows:

1. Control/precision
2. Multi-limb co-ordination
3. Response orientation
4. Reaction time
5. Speed of arm movements
6. Rate control (timing)
7. Manual dexterity
8. Finger dexterity
9. Hand–arm steadiness
10. Wrist/finger movement/speed

All of these attributes can be identified during patient lifting when the arms, hands and legs of the lifter have to move in a co-ordinated fashion, reactive to the needs of the situation as it changes.

CURRICULAR ISSUES AFFECTING LEVEL OF APPROACH

Curricula should be developed and planned with the following issues in mind (after Tyler 1949).

1. What is the educational purpose of the course/training?
2. What experiences can be provided to meet this purpose?

3. How can the experience be organised?

4. How can we determine that the purposes are being attained?

The educational purpose of the curriculum for a course is to achieve a certain level of learning. The correct level is crucial to the students' success. The level in a curriculum is confirmed by the assessment process, the broad direction of the content often being similar to other courses. For example, lifting and moving can be taught to anyone from portering staff to relatives who are carers in the home, to students of nursing, midwifery and physiotherapy. The intended level of teaching and learning for all of these is clearly different.

For the porter, you would teach safe and comfortable lifting and moving techniques of both objects and patients/clients and assess him or her on the technical accuracy of the procedure, a key issue being that he does harm to neither the patient nor himself.

For the home carer, you would need also to teach how to adapt resources for lifting and assessment would be based on grounds of safety for both parties and would be on an informal basis.

For the student nurse or midwife, not only would comfort be involved but prevention and relief of pressure, the hazards of immobility, how to prevent positional deformity, how to gain the patient's/client's co-operation and so on. You would also teach the background to the physiological aspects of movements, related to the musculo-skeletal system. The student would be assessed formally on how well these aspects had been integrated. Assessment would also focus on the student's ability to communicate with the patient/client and to predict the consequences of poor technique.

For the physiotherapy student, the teacher would need to include all the points described for the student nurse or midwife, plus more detail on the role of the musculo-skeletal system. Assessment would also be formal and include prediction of problems. In this instance, the physiotherapy student may also be required to prescribe treatment to facilitate movement, in terms of appropriate exercises.

No matter what the level of the teaching, the practitioner-teacher needs to know what knowledge the student already has and to be able to determine if this knowledge is accurate. The teacher then has to determine the level the student has to reach and the content required to get the student there.

Teaching Students of Mixed Ability

Having determined the level and the content of the material to be taught, it is necessary to select the best strategy to teach it. This will depend on the learning style of the student and his or her learning curve, the content to be delivered and the teacher's preferred method.

For example, some people learn better by discussion followed by demonstration, and others by mostly demonstration followed by description. This will depend on their learning style. With regard to learning curves, some people will learn a particular skill in a relatively short period of time, whilst it will take others much longer, with no resulting difference in competence in the final outcome.

The content to be delivered should be presented appropriately, making best use of all resources available to the teacher, ensuring clarity of presentation and avoiding any potential ambiguities. Remember that visual information is better retained than oral information and that actually doing something is the best way of learning.

The teacher's ability is also crucial as to how a topic should be presented. For example, if the teacher is less sure of him or herself when leading discussion groups, it may be better to get the group to present information in a seminar.

The process model for curriculum design (described by Stenhouse 1975) is useful to enable accomplishment by people of different ability levels.

The process model can be seen as more to do with education than training, with a strong focus on developing understanding. The process model demands an active role of the student; the teacher assumes the role of **facilitator**. It affords a student-centred approach, allowing the student to develop their own skills at their own pace.

There are no set objectives to achieve by specific time-scales. There are outcomes which can be attained over a longer period and the method of reaching the outcome allows for individual student differences. The process model involves experience rather than instruction and is well suited to the needs and abilities of adult learners.

For simple tasks, a product model which focuses on the completion of the end-product of learning rather than the process may be appropriate since straightforward instruction may be what is needed to pass on information of a safety nature. For example, when teaching students of different abilities, the teacher must assess the needs of each individual student, and define the process each must go through to reach the desired outcomes, and decide the teacher activities to facilitate the student's learning.

Regardless of ability, students will need to achieve competence in the clinical area where the teaching and learning is taking place. The practitioner-teacher must ensure that the student follows an appropriate route to achieving competence.

Activity 4.6.

Think of a skill you might teach to a student.

Think why it is realistic to expect him or her to learn this.

State the expected outcome(s).

Identify how the skill is capable of being demonstrated, observed and assessed. State how it relates to other skills the student needs to acquire.

Describe how the student can demonstrate his or her ability to perform the skill.

Determine if the student has got the necessary manual dexterity, knowledge or other personal attributes which may be needed.

Thus, in helping a student to achieve competence, you need to be certain that the thing to be learned:

- is realistic
- has clearly accomplishable outcomes
- is capable of demonstration, observation, assessment
- relates to other skills either learned in the past or to be learned in the future
- is appropriate to the student's existing knowledge and skills.

Practical Teaching Considerations Related to Problems of Adjusting Levels

The teacher should make it her business to ascertain the students' needs and ensure that they are taught at the relevant level.

Teachers may find difficulties with teaching the same subject to various students all at different levels. There is an additional problem if this occurs several times a day with the same subject! It is useful consciously to switch off after any teaching session so that you tackle the next one with a fresh approach. For example, you may have been teaching a student nurse how to give an injection and in the next half hour have to show ten year old Johnnie how to give himself insulin injections. You will obviously need very different approaches and strategies for the two sessions, and in order to avoid interference from the previous session, you must mentally switch off between the two periods of teaching.

Teacher Expectations

There are certain expectations about the role of the teacher, both on the part of the institution within which he is teaching and on the part of the student. Hargreaves (1972) compiled a picture of what school children in the UK expected teachers to be like, and although we are not talking here about teaching school children, nevertheless the traits seen as desirable are likely to be applicable to teachers of nursing and midwifery students.

Children tend to like	*Children tend to dislike*
A teacher who	A teacher who . . . .

(1 Discipline)

keeps good control	is too strict, too lax,
is fair, has no favourites	has favourites, picks on pupils,
gives no extreme or immoderate punishments	punishes and threatens excessively/arbitrarily

(2 Instruction)

explains and helps	doesn't explain,
gives interesting lessons	gives little help,
	does not know subject well,
	gives dull or boring lessons

(3 Personality)

is cheerful, friendly, patient, understanding, etc.	nags, ridicules, is sarcastic, bad-tempered, unkind, etc.
has a good sense of humour	has no sense of humour
takes an interest in pupils as individuals.	ignores individual differences.

These characteristics can easily be applied to any teacher with any student. Whilst the research focused on children, the overriding principle that stands out is respect for persons. Respect for persons is integrated into most educational and caring philosophies nowadays and applies equally to persons of all ages, in all situations, and is an expectation of the teacher.

There is strong evidence to show that the teacher can determine the nature of the student interaction in terms of power relationships. French and Raven (1959) in Glen (1975) described bases of power in organisations as follows:

Reward Power   —ensure compliance with those who can give or
                  withhold rewards
Coercive Power   —power to punish non-compliance
Expert Power   —the possession of knowledge which is in demand
Referent Power   —power associated with popularity
Legitimate Power—where the organisational structure confers it

The culture within which the practitioner-teacher operates allows for
Expert Power and Referent Power as appropriate. It also allows for Legitimate Power in relation to student nurses and midwives.

CONCLUSION

Note that material in this chapter on differences in learning styles enhan-
ces that presented on assessing learning needs in chapter 2. Similarly,
teaching a skill, which is addressed in chapter 3: *Planning for Teaching*,
is approached here from the viewpoint of differences in ability. Chapter 3
additionally focuses on planning to teach a topic at a range of levels; here
the emphasis has been on the use of a process or product approach within
differing strategies.

   This chapter has attempted to give you an insight into the many sociological, physiological and curricular factors which affect the teaching
process for the practitioner-teacher and student. The interrelationships
are complex, and the practitioner as teacher should familiarise herself
with all the factors in order to increase his or her effectiveness.

   If, in your teaching, you are able to focus on differences in your students
to do with their language, culture, peer group relationships and learning
styles, you will be in a position to maximise your teaching.

GLOSSARY

Accent: a national local or individual way of pronouncing words.

Culture: the customs and civilisation of a particular group of people,
including such aspects as dietary habits, art, dance, dress and religion.

Dialect: the words and pronunciation used in a particular area of a
country.

Facilitator: one who enables. Thus, the teacher, when acting as a facilitator, manages the teaching situation so that learning is most likely to
occur. The approach is generally regarded as being student-centred with
the teacher helping the student to explore and use all the resources
available.

Peer group: a group of people who are associated and of equal status, usually sharing a common approach to dress, language, values, recreation, etc. The group to whom one relates, from whom one may derive values.

Sub-culture: a group within a culture sharing the same patterns of belief, behaviour, attitudes and values and distinguishable form the overall culture of the society.

REFERENCES

Bernstein B (1962) Linguistic Codes, Hesitation Phenomena and Intelligence. *Language and Speech*, **5**, Jan–March.

Bernstein B (1960) Language and Social Class. *British Journal of Sociology*, **11**.

Bruner J S (1974) *Relevance of Education*. London: Penguin.

Glen F (1975) The Social Psychology of Organisations, in Peter Herriot, *Essential Psychology*. London: Methuen.

Hargreaves P H (1972) *Interpersonal Relations and Education*. London: Routledge and Kegan Paul.

Labo W (1970) The Study of Language in its Social Context. *Studium Generale*, **23**(1).

Mead G H (1934) *Mind, Self and Society*. Chicago: University of Chicago Press.

Merton R K (1957) *Social Theory and Social Structure*. Chicago: The Free Press of Glencoe.

Stenhouse L (1975) *An Introduction to Curriculum Research and Development* (Chapter 7). London: Heinemann.

Thomas A and Chess S (1977) *Temperament and Development*. New York: Bruner/Mazel.

Tyler R W (1949) *Basic Principles of Curriculum and Instruction*. Chicago: University of Chicago Press.

Wharf B L (1956) Science and Linguistics, in J B Carroll (Ed) *Language Thought and Reality: selected writings of Benjamin Lee Wharfe*. Cambridge MA: MIT Press.

Wittgenstein L (1953) *Philosophical Investigations*. Oxford: Blackwell and translated by G E M Anscombe, New York: Macmillan.

SUGGESTIONS FOR FURTHER READING

Andrews J (1984) *Understanding Sociology*. Surrey: Nelson. This is a basic text, providing a clear and easy to read introduction to sociology. You will need to make your own links between the general information contained here on sociology and its application to teaching.

Atkinson R L, Atkinson R C, Smith E E, Bem D J and Hildegarde E R (1990) *Introduction to Psychology* (10th edn). New York: Harcourt Brace Jovnovich. A classic undergraduate psychology textbook, it gives the student an excellent introduction to psychology, is easy to read and well illustrated.

Daws J (1988) An Inquiry into the Attitudes of Qualified Nursing Staff towards the Use of Individualised Nursing Care Plans as a Teaching Tool. *Journal of Advanced Nursing*, **13**, 139–146. A study of the approach practitioners take to implementing change and the lessons this holds for teachers.

Hirst P H and Peters R S (1970) *The Logic of Education*, London: Routledge and Kegan Paul. This is a classic text and an Open University set book. It gives the student a background to the philosophy of education, the aims of education, how people learn and an introduction to curriculum development.

Rogers C (1983) *Freedom to Learn in the 80's*. Columbus, Ohio: Charles Merrill. Many Colleges of Nursing base their philosophies of education on Carl Rogers' original work, of which this is an extension. His humanist perspective translates easily from student nurses to patients or indeed to anyone you may have to teach. It would be very useful to familiarise yourself with this text.

Sheahan J (1981) Developing Teaching Skills. *Nursing Focus* (November) **3**(3), 543–547. A useful article on teaching skills, suitable for practitioners.

Chapter 5

Evaluating Your Teaching:
Are Your Goals Being Met?

INTRODUCTION

In the opening chapter of this book, several of the activities you were urged to undertake included an evaluation of your actions. Using a systematic approach to care with your patients or clients, you will be familiar with evaluating the care given, and goals will have been established in order for you to evaluate the outcomes. Transferral of this skill to evaluation of your teaching in clinical practice will, for some, already have occurred, whilst others are likely to require additional help in this area. Whichever of these descriptions applies to you, it is envisaged that this chapter will provide additional useful information on the skills of evaluating your teaching.

With the current thrust towards Quality Assurance, most clinical areas are developing or have developed 'standards', and nursing and midwifery education is no exception. Standard-setting and its place in teaching practitioners, patients, clients and relatives will be explored, together with advice on analysis of situations prior to suitable standards being set. Balogh, Beattie and Beckerleg (1989) suggest that we cannot evaluate without using some pre-defined criteria.

The word 'evaluation' can mean different things to different people. This chapter aims to help you develop not only your own workable standards but also your own personal definition of evaluation and how it fits into the setting in which you work. What you have learned from the evaluation of practice should be used as a baseline to aid this development. To help you achieve this, there will be some discussion on the similarities and differences between evaluation of care and evaluation of teaching.

The need for clarity about exactly what is to be evaluated, and how this is to be done will be emphasised. Empirical research, psychometric testing and illuminative approaches to evaluation will be discussed.

Once evaluation has taken place it is easy to assume that the process of teaching is complete. However, evaluation can only be effective if something is actually done with the information acquired. Suggestions on how to bring about any necessary changes are included.

Activity 5.1.

Write down what the term evaluation means to you. Initially make no attempt to order your thoughts on this, simply write down whatever comes into your head.

Now follow this through by attempting to write down your own definition of the word 'evaluation'.

The English National Board for Nursing Midwifery and Health Visiting give the following definition of evaluation:

'the collection and use of information in order to make decisions about an educational programme.'

Wheeler (1970) states that to understand evaluation there is a need to differentiate between evaluation, assessment and measurement. You may have used such words as assessment, measurement and monitoring, checking, reflecting, in your definition of the word evaluation. Evaluation can include some or all of these points. Wheeler defines evaluations as outcomes based on judgement of change, and stresses the importance of assessment as a prerequisite to evaluation.

You may think of evaluation as something which takes place at the end of a course or a study day, and indeed the ENB's definition tends to indicate that this is so. But this is only one type of evaluation, which is usually referred to as *summative*.

Bradshaw (1989) defines evaluation in the context of the nursing process as: 'appraisal of the outcome'. He comments that this can represent either a satisfactory conclusion of care or show that care may have been ineffective. Such a clearcut evaluation is unlikely to occur in practice, either as an evaluation of care or teaching. In general, evaluations tend to show a mixture of good and bad points and obviously it is more encouraging to

both learner and teacher to focus on positive aspects. Indeed, it is important that learners continue to develop and enhance their potential.
However, areas where improvement is necessary need clear and constructive advice if practice is to benefit.

As a teacher-practitioner, evaluation of the learning that has been
achieved as a result of your actions ought to be part of your everyday
thinking. This ongoing or diagnostic evaluation is described as *formative*.
Evaluation of both teaching and practice will show positive and, inevit-
ably, sometimes negative aspects. It is by the recognition of and reflection
on both positive and negative features that we can improve our practice.

Sometimes, in performing an evaluation, a scale of measurement may be
used against which the expected goals or outcomes can be rated. These
expected goals must have previously been set, together with criteria for
assessing achievement. Lawton (1983) suggests that the factors to be assessed and measured as part of a curriculum include 'not only what is
taught but how it is taught and why'. To the teacher-practitioner, this can
at first appear to be a rather complex view, so it is worthwhile spending
some time producing a structure whereby goals can easily be set and their
achievement be measured.

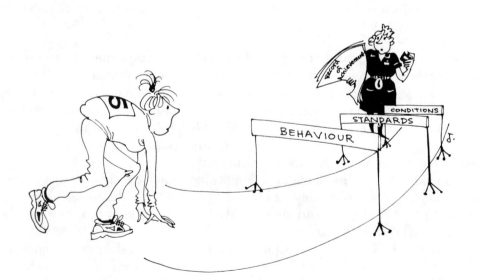

1. SETTING THE STRUCTURE

1.1. Goal Setting

Narrow (1979) states that 'evaluation is easy if the standards or criteria are objective and precise'. The terminology used can vary: behavioural objectives, outcomes, goals, standards or criteria, and all have a different emphasis. The descriptive noun used usually depends on the purpose of the activity and the organisation involved. Whilst nurse and midwifery education, in some areas, is moving away from behavioural objectives and towards outcomes, nursing and midwifery management is tending to follow business management, and thus the defining of standards and criteria.

1.2. Behavioural Objectives

During the last two decades much emphasis has been placed on the writing of behavioural objectives. Mager (1984) suggests that the purpose of using behavioural objectives is to ensure, on evaluation, that the following three questions are answered:

1.   What should the learner be able to do? (the behaviour).

2.   How well should he be able to do it? (the criteria).

3.   Under what conditions should he be able to do it? (the condition).

Activity 5.1.2.

Using the above three questions, think of a teaching/learning situation that you are familiar with in your area of work and write down a list of behavioural objectives.

Applying this concept to a task-orientated activity such as taking the body temperature of a baby, these are some of the points you might consider:

1.   The learner should be able to use an electronic thermometer to record the core temperature of the baby.

2.   The learner should be able to do this accurately. This entails
      —ensuring the battery to the machine is charged

—using the correct disposable sheaths for the metal probe.
—placing the probe in the correct position
—correctly reading and recording the figure shown on the electronic display

3. Your student might be new to the clinical situation, so the conditions under which you would expect her to carry out the activity would differ from those of an experienced practitioner. 'Under guidance' or 'under supervision' are words you would use to describe the conditions under which the activity might occur.

By breaking down any activity into component parts you can begin its analysis. In a day-to-day situation you are unlikely to consider each teaching opportunity in this way. The example is used here as a means of reflection, serving to emphasise what you are expecting someone in a learning situation to achieve.

Bloom et al (1981) state that learning can be classified into three domains, namely

cognitive
psychomotor
affective.

The *cognitive* domain appertains to the knowledge gained, e.g. about the physiology of the heart, or differing psychological theories of learning.

The *psychomotor* domain refers to the gaining of a skill, e.g. bathing a baby, or communicating effectively with a client with learning difficulties.

The *affective* domain signifies changes in attitudinal behaviour, e.g. the new entrant to nursing may believe that all abortions are wrong; professional education can provide different perspectives on the situation, with a subsequent modification of attitude.

Behavioural objectives tend to relate mainly to the psychomotor domain, but the application of knowledge to practice can demonstrate learning in the cognitive domain. For example, a student may demonstrate that she is able to take a person's pulse and record her findings. The same student takes a person's pulse, observes that the individual is pale and clammy, understands that the pulse is not within normal limits and that this may signify internal bleeding. When the student takes appropriate action by informing the nurse or midwife in charge, there is adequate evidence to assume that the student has applied knowledge to practice, thus demonstrating knowledge in the cognitive domain.

Andrusyszyn (1989) suggests that changes in the affective domain are more difficult to measure or evaluate, e.g. an individual may deny they are racially prejudiced but discover, with **experiential learning** and open discussion, that they exhibit some behaviour indicative of discrimination. Andrusyszyn cites Litwak (1979) who comments on page 75 that:

> 'Clinical evaluation is the most important dimension in the process of evaluating student learning and mastery. The process consists of evaluating students' abilities to integrate cognitive, affective, and psychomotor skills when delivering nursing care.'

The paper by Andrusyszyn provides a well-balanced discussion of evaluation of the affective domain and it is well worth reading.

1.3. Needs Analysis

Harris and Bell (1986) refer to the drawing up of criteria for evaluation purposes prior to learning as 'needs analysis'. In an era of student-centred learning, where students are encouraged to define their own needs, it is important that teacher and practitioner work together. Burnard (1990) highlights the incongruence of placing the emphasis on learning which is student-initiated with curricula focused heavily on theoretical content. The teacher-practitioner needs to be aware of the factors which are desirable as well as necessary to aid learning. Harris and Bell (1986) suggest

---

Activity 5.1.3.

Get together wtih a group of colleagues, choose a subject area common to you all and individually write answers to these three questions:

— what do I need to learn?
— what do I want to learn?
— how may I best learn?

Now discuss your answers. Did you find that you all chose exactly the same aspects of the subject, as areas you may need or want to learn?

Did you notice any differences between that which you wanted to learn and that which you knew you ought to learn?

---

that learners must ask themselves: 'What do I need to learn? What do I want to learn? How may I best learn?'

The third question undoubtedly will have provoked different ideas of how you best learn. The same applies to those whom you are teaching. To apply the needs analysis concept, each learner ought to be encouraged to ask themselves similar questions in order to decide the criteria for their goals.

Assuming that the purpose of evaluation is solely to enhance teaching and thus learning, it will be relevant to match the needs of the student and their learning styles with the method of teaching. It is only by the teacher asking appropriate questions within the evaluation process that this can be achieved. In this case, the teacher and learner both need the information.

The learning content will vary from learner to learner and this will be dependent on whether the content is learner- or teacher-initiated and whether the teaching method matches the students' preferred learning style. Armitage and Burnard (1991) point out that although there has been movement towards student-centred learning in nurse education, there are several studies to suggest that the students themselves would often prefer a more structured, didactic style of teaching (Burnard 1990, Spouse 1990, Armitage and Burnard 1991). Harris and Bell (1986) stress that all individuals are different and in every case the previous knowledge and

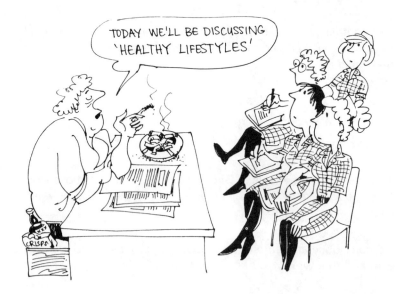

personal background of the individual will affect the degree of learning that takes place.

A good starting point for all learners is to relate to something with which they are familiar. For example, during a health promotion session with either student or client, a discussion on healthy eating habits will cause the learner to focus on their own habits, and those of other people they know. The content of this type of session is relatively easy to pursue; facts can be imparted, but the sharing, adaptation and changing of personal habits is a less easy aspect on which to dwell. Whilst the practitioner may find a patient or client who needs to alter her eating pattern for health reasons is likely to be amenable to change, the student who considers herself healthy may be less open to change.

2. MEASURING PERFORMANCES

2.1. Standards and Performance Indicators

In order to help clarify expected goals, it is useful to consider the 'standards' that have been set in your area of practice. Not all clinical areas have completed the setting of standards, so it is worthwhile taking some time to explore this subject. Spouse (1990) discusses 'performance indicators' as an indication of an expected standard. On page 42 she states that: 'Performance Indicators enable the collection of data that permit identification of quantitative and qualitative values of activities to be made.' She uses the word 'permit' in relation to the identification of effective resources and suggests that performance indicators can be used to encourage an input of resources. Once standards have been set, performance indicators can be used as a tool to establish whether or not the standards have been met.

2.2. Standards

Although the purpose of setting standards within the clinical area is not primarily geared towards education, at least one of the 'standards' devised in your area of work will relate to the learner and the learning environment. Standards and quality go hand in hand, and, following extensive research, Alison Kitson spearheaded the development of a teaching pack, published by the Royal College of Nursing in 1990. This pack is listed amongst the suggestions for further reading, and provides interesting, easy to follow explanations and discussions on setting standards using a Dynamic Standard Setting System framework. If the teacher as practitioner takes advantage of set standards related to learning, she will be able to utilise them for the benefit of both teacher and learner.

Returning to the work of Spouse, she aimed to build on the research into the clinical learning environment undertaken by Fretwell (1982 and 1985), Ogier (1982), Orton (1981) and Reid (1985). Spouse applied the guidelines suggested by Donabedian (1966) as a framework for the formulation of standards and discusses how standards can set the scene for the ward learning climate. She describes how standards can be devised using the three interlinked areas of outcomes, structure and process as proposed by Donabedian.

Outcomes

The desired learning outcomes for students of nursing or midwifery and can be planned by:

1. Educationalists and clinicians as part of the curriculum for a total course or a part of a course,

2. Clinicians as teachers, with or without student negotiation, but preferably together with the student,

3. Clinicians in negotiation with patients/clients.

Process

Process describes the organisation and implementation of the planned outcomes. The process element is concerned with asking questions and finding appropriate answers. How will the outcome be achieved? Who will achieve it? What are the resources that will be involved? For instance, for a student on a clinical placement, the following are examples of areas that may be considered under the process heading:

1. The student's participation/contribution to planning individualised patient/client care.

2. The strategies used by practitioners to include the student in the care of patients and clients.

3. The methods used to facilitate opportunities for students gaining additional experience related to their given area of work, i.e. their exposure to learning situations.

4. The type of ward management in a given situation, i.e. whether it is task-orientated, patient-allocation, team-nursing/midwifery or primary nursing or midwifery care.

5. The amount of time the student spends with a registered practitioner.

6. The use of learning contracts, diaries, logs, journals or other methods of providing a planned record of student progress.

Structure

Many of the activities within the outcome and process sections are dependant on the structure of the organisation and the policies therein. The method of management of a clinical area may be linked with the number of staff available and the skill-mix involved. All Health Authorities preparing to implement Project 2000 from April 1990 were directed to consider and alter their 'skill mix' (Department of Health Communications 1989/1990). This is due to the fact that Project 2000 students will not be counted as part of the workforce. Guidelines for the type of skill mix are, however, limited. All skilled practitioners, faced with the choice of employing trained staff or health care support workers, may find it useful to consider Spouse's following suggestions. She believes that for a clinical area to be considered as suitable for student teaching the following points are useful to consider:

• level one nurses should be appointed who are able to demonstrate an interest in their own professional development and the teaching of others.

• the availability of ongoing post-basic education for all level one nurses together with the opportunity for attendance. Theoretically this should be made easier following the implementation of the Post Registration Education and Practice Project (PREPP 1990) recommendations in 1991.

• the content and quality of orientation programmes for staff and students new to the clinical area.

• the availability and accessibility of learning experiences to students.

This is usually elucidated from the educational audit carried out by Colleges of Nursing and Midwifery prior to allocation of learners to specific areas. Many Project 2000 training and education programmes have now made it compulsory for students to visit other departments within a hospital to study the full range of practice areas. As this is a major change in the training and education of students of nursing, there is a necessity for its formal recognition. Ward managers and nurses in charge of clinical areas should be aware that future students cannot be considered as a constant source of labour in clinical areas; furthermore, they will require additional support and teaching, in order to ensure that the experience they have is relevant to the provision of care for the patient/client.

2.3. Performance Indicators

To give you some ideas of what performance indicators are and what they are not, try to read the English National Board guide 'Figuring out performance' compiled by Balogh, Beattie and Beckerleg (1989). This document devotes several pages to the concept of performance indicators, but ultimately gives no definition, or cut and dried rule in relation to them. Performance indicators are described by Balogh et al on page 8 as:

- 'guides rather than absolute measures'

- 'having numerical values which assess aspects of a system'.

The gathering of data to measure performance in relation to a standard often will result in the collection of numbers. In industry and business, where performance indicators originated, it is relatively easy to count the number of items of a product that have been sold, or the number of staff employed. In nursing and midwifery, whilst it is relatively easy to transfer this concept to the counting of staff and those starting and leaving employment, it is less easy to envisage numerical values in relation to patient or client care. However, one example of its application could be counting the number of formal teaching sessions in a clinical area, and in addition, some attempt be made to evaluate their success.

Performance indicators can only be set once standards have been defined. For the teacher-practitioner, working in the clinical area, performance indicators are more likely to be set in order to measure the total performance of the nursing team, and are less likely to suggest a suitable method for evaluation of an individual teaching activity. Standards, on the other hand, aim to ensure quality both in care and education. Performance indicators can be said to deal with the monitoring and measurement of results achieved after an activity has taken place, whereas the setting of standards is a prerequisite.

Activity 5.2.3.

Assume your area of work has set the following standard:

'There is a clear strategy for effective oral and written communication between all personnel.'

1. Write down your ideas of how this might be achieved.

2. Write down how you will monitor that these criteria have been achieved, i.e. you will be writing down your performance indicators.

You will probably have thought about oral and written reports and given some consideration to the methods used for recording and passing on information. This should not be merely amongst nursing and midwifery personnel but should include all members of the multidisciplinary team, patients/clients and their relatives. Your performance indicators could encompass some record of numbers of successful or unsuccessful communications. Effective teaching encounters could also be included. Remember there are no right and wrong indicators as these will differ with your personal situation.

3. EVALUATING ONGOING LEARNING

The learning/teaching process should be an active two-way communication system. Ideally questions and answers should flow freely between learner and teacher. Whilst the teacher needs to question to ascertain what the learner already understands, the learner must be able to question to clarify areas of which she is uncertain. Both teacher and pupil throughout this process will be assessing independently the learning which is taking place. The teacher will be able to identify where the student is having difficulty, by reading the cues provided by the student, for example a puzzled expression, or body language indicating boredom. The tone of voice used in discussion and questioning by both parties will also indicate their interest, rapport and give some evidence of the learning that is taking place.

One of the simplest forms of ongoing evaluation is that of simple discussion between learner and teacher. The method of teaching can be discussed before the teaching encounter, during the session or at any other time agreeable to both parties. Harris and Bell (1986) claim that such discussions 'reduce alienation and ensure motivation'.

Activity 5.3.1.

Think of a teaching session that you have recently given or attended as a student. Enumerate the ways in which students provided cues to the teacher about their state of motivation, interest or attention.

It is likely that you came up with a number of examples in addition to:

- looking out of the window
- chatting
- yawning
- looking glazed

With practice you should be able to decrease such instances occurring in your own sessions!

4.   DIFFERENT METHODS OF PLANNING FOR EVALUATION

Regardless of the type of objective, outcome or standard that you are working towards, a judgement has to be made, when evaluating, as to whether or not the criteria set have been achieved.

The checklist provided by Harris and Bell (1986) to aid forward planning has here been modified. Perhaps after using it in the following activity you will be able to adapt and modify it further for your own purposes and use it in addition to the set criteria.

Activity 5.4.1.

Think of a teaching session that you are due to give within the next month and ask yourself

---

continued on next page

continued

— What do I hope to achieve?

— How can the important issues be identified?

— Whom do I need to negotiate with?

— How will I ensure rapport and communication are maintained?

— How will I collect and analyse information in order to evaluate the session?

— Who will be interested in the findings from the evaluation?

— Am I the best person to collect the information or do I need to involve someone else? If so, who?

— Who will give me the information I require in order to carry out the evaluation? Is it solely a student of nursing or midwifery, or are patients/clients or other members of the multidisciplinary team involved?

If you have had some difficulty in answering these questions, use the following scenario as a guide.

John Brownlow, a 76 year old gentleman, has spent several weeks in hospital because his wife is unable to cope with his increasing dementia. His son and his wife are willing to take John to live with them. They ask for additional information to help them cope with the aggressive periods of dementia from which John suffers.

Your answers to the previous questions cited in the activity may be as follows:

You hope to give John's relatives sufficient information to boost their confidence, to the benefit of all concerned. Important issues can be identified by discussing with John's wife and his son and daughter-in-law the specific points that are worrying them. You would be able to refer to the record of John's care whilst in hospital to determine, potential problem areas, and instigate tried and tested solutions. Other professionals such as the Community Psychiatric Nurse and Social Worker may need to be involved in the negotiations and discussions. In order to ensure that rapport and communication are maintained, dates and times will need to be negotiated with John's relatives for appropriate information sessions. Their previous knowledge will need to be ascertained and you will need to use your own judgement to help you to select suitable communication techniques.

Evaluating your planned teaching strategies will require you not only to ask John's relatives relevant questions, but also to arrange follow-up support, to judge the effectiveness of the proposed methods of care. You may also ask yourself questions in order to determine the degree of success of each teaching encounter, e.g. Were there any cues to indicate boredom or misunderstanding from the relatives? Were the relatives able to answer any questions you asked to ascertain their previous knowledge or understanding? Did John's relatives ask you questions? In the example given, the evaluation will affect you as the teacher, the relatives and John as recipients of proposed actions, and the Community Psychiatric Nurse and Social Worker as their roles expand or diminish. There will certainly be a need, in this case, to involve others in the evaluation and the question of whom this should be has already been addressed.

Bradshaw (1989) suggests examples for a self-evaluation checklist for clinical supervisors. Many of these are pertinent to the teacher-practitioner. Look through the list below which is adapted from page 111 of Bradshaw's book *Teaching and Assessing in Clinical Nursing Practice* and reflect on them in relation to your area of clinical teaching.

1. Do I read the nursing press regularly and discuss current professional issues with colleagues?

2. Am I up-to-date with publications, developments and research in my specialist field?

3. Do I attend continuing education events of both a general and specialist nature, e.g. courses, conferences, seminars?

4. Do I make full use of professional library resources?

5. Have I visited other centres specialising in my branch of nursing?

6. Do I have a personal philosophy for care delivery?

7. Is my philosophy consistent with current expectations for nursing or midwifery practice?

8. Is my philosophy evident in my practice?

9. Do I have a commitment to offer professional development to junior colleagues?

10. Do I assess their learning needs adequately and attempt to meet these?

This list should provoke thought about how your practice can be improved. It is not exhaustive and doesn't even begin to look at the actual evaluation of teaching, but it should give you the opportunity to reflect on your own practice without specifically focusing on a given situation.

Do try to read Spouse's research (1990) into the clinical learning environment. It is interesting to see evaluation from the differing perspectives of students, qualified practitioners as teachers and educationalists. Indeed, the opinion of the qualified nurse or nurse teacher may be at variance with that of the student, in relation to what constitutes a suitable environment for learning. This work is supported by that of Marson (1982) who noted that the emphasis and importance placed on various aspects of the learning situation differed between learner, ward sister and nurse tutor. Whilst there was some agreement regarding relevant factors, the differences were in the priority placed on individual components. Spouse, Marson, Mogan and Knox (1987) found that learners put much greater emphasis on the importance of the teacher being approachable, fostering mutual respect, demonstrating enthusiasm and correcting them without belittlement than on the quality of the teaching itself. Marson found that above 80 per cent of student and pupil nurses completing her questionnaire thought that the characteristics of good teaching included, not only displaying high standards of care and setting good examples, but also demonstrating care and concern for patient's/client's needs and having time for trainees.

Later in the chapter, when you come to devise your own evaluation criteria, remember to take into consideration the above research on the learning environment. For this, you might like to consider SWOT Analysis, i.e. examining the Strengths, Weaknesses, Opportunities and Threats of a particular situation. This is a concept taken from business planning and management, which is rapidly flooding the health arena. Selective use of *Marketing Management: Analysis, Planning, Implementation and Control* by Philip Kotler (1988) can provide additional inspiration for the highly motivated.

There are times, within the clinical area when you may find yourself in an unexpected teaching situation, that is, an unplanned, natural opportunity to teach either patient, relative or learners. Hinchliff (1986) calls this 'crisis teaching'. Successful teaching, in this situation, probably only takes place due to the practitioner's expertise and knowledge in the given area, but evaluation of the teaching experience, as soon as it is practicable to the management of the ward, or client situation can enhance learning and provide valuable information for future occasions. Benner (1984) provides descriptive examples of situations where there is a need for immediate action or teaching. There is much evidence in Benner's work to support the notion that the advanced or expert practitioner has more to offer than the less experienced.

Activity 5.4.2.

Think of an instance when you have been called upon to teach in an unplanned, spontaneous way.

1. Was it successful? If not, why not? If it was successful, why do you think this was so?

2. Considering the answers you gave in 1, write down how you think you could improve unplanned teaching sessions in the future.

In an emergency situation the experienced nurse (Benner's 'expert practitioner') deals with the problem in hand and at the same time manages other personnel, giving out instructions. The rationale for what she is doing may or may not be given at this time. The learner should be motivated, following the incident, to ask questions and seek information. It is then the role of the expert practitioner to clarify the situation, and Hinchliff argues that it is not too late at this stage to set objectives and work to a planned framework.

Models of Evaluation

It is useful here to examine some models of evaluation as identified by Kenworthy and Nicklin (1989). Although these are intended primarily as strategies for course evaluations, it is worthwhile to extrapolate from them the factors which are pertinent to the individual intent on evaluating whether this is the students themselves or their teacher.

4.1. Classical experimental model

This model uses behavioural objectives as a framework of criteria for measuring achievement. Take as an example the giving of an injection by a student nurse or the self-administration of an injection by a diabetic patient or client. Using the classical evaluation model, this skill would be broken down into small component parts and the emphasis would be on whether the achievement of each of these could be demonstrated. Less easily quantifiable factors, such as the patient's/client's acceptance of diabetes mellitus, or the practitioner's rapport and empathy with that patient are not readily assessed by this method; however, competence within the psychomotor or cognitive domains can be recognised, i.e. the skill of giving an injection is a psychomotor one, but background knowledge is also required. Knowledge relates to the cognitive domain, whilst rapport and empathy relate to the affective domain.

A further example of the differences between the three domains can be identified by examining the act of bottle-feeding a baby. The mother, nurse or midwife requires prior knowledge of the correct feed to give, and the correct method of administration (cognitive domain) and whilst implementing this activity can show psychomotor dexterity. The element of providing warm, confident comfort whilst holding the baby is not easy to observe and can be perhaps classified within the affective domain. Look again at the above examples and carry out the following activity.

Activity 5.4.3.

Together with a colleague or group of fellow students draw up:

(i) a list of learning situations which mainly involve psychomotor and cognitive skills, which you believe could be evaluated by measuring the learner's achievement of behavioural objectives.

(ii) a list of competencies within the affective domain which you think are less easily measurable by behavioural objectives.

Was the task easy? Was it cut and dried? Or did you disagree about certain points?

Learning is a complex process, and the text aims throughout to impress upon you that there are no right and wrong answers, but hopefully you will be provided with 'food for thought' and sufficient interest and motivation to help you improve your practice and that of others.

4.2. The illuminative model (Anthropological model)

The Anthropological model refers to a method of evaluation with wider perspectives, and is in contrast to evaluations which look at solely quantitative factors. Anthropology looks at the science of man from both psychological and physiological perspectives and thus the emphasis in this model is on description and interpretation based on observation and interview. The emphasis here is on **qualitative** factors, and the opinions of the participants and observers of a teaching encounter are considered. Descriptions and individual interpretations of the situation are taken into account in order to provide an apt evaluation. For example, considering the client with an obsessive disorder, it may not be easy to elucidate the degree of modification in the patient's behaviour that has been achieved; using the illuminative approach, several people's opinions can be sought and interviews with both nurse and client would be undertaken before conclusions were drawn. It can be argued, however, that this type of evaluation can be too subjective and open to bias.

4.3. The briefing decision-maker's model (sometimes referred to as the 'political' model)

Here an external evaluator looks at a given situation, and passes their opinion on to those 'in authority'. Although this is more likely to produce an unbiased opinion, it is an option only open in a limited number of situations. Unless a full-length research study was in progress, within the clinical situation there is usually little time or funding to pursue such a course. Further discussion of this model is outside the remit of the book and readers are advised to refer to Kenworthy and Nicklin (1989) for further information about this interesting aspect of evaluation.

4.4. The teacher as a researcher model

This is probably the type of evaluation with which you are most familiar, as you yourself may have been asked to complete evaluation forms at the end of a course, unit or study day. As Colleges of Nursing and Midwifery aim to meet their mission statements, the emphasis on this kind of evaluation is becoming more pronounced. For those unfamiliar with the term 'mission statement' this is a statement of intent usually focused on the business plans for an institution for a period of time from one to three years. This statement is updated annually and allows planning for the future. For example, the mission statement for nursing or midwifery managers could be to ensure that all patients/clients receive appropriate care, at a suitable time, safely delivered by trained practitioners.

4.5. The case-study model

This incorporates both qualitative and **quantitative** factors, using a combination of questionnaires to match objectives, together with observation and the seeking of opinions from a variety of people. In many ways this model can be compared with the briefing decision-maker's model. Kenworthy and Nicklin (1989) point out that both models usually involve an external assessor and are therefore costly to implement. They suggest that the case-study model is more likely to be used to confirm a decision that has already been made.

4.6. Questionnaires

Questionnaires can be designed to focus on material learnt, the learning environment, the quality of the teaching, the quantity and quality of the theoretical content, or the relevance of the theory to the situation. Questionnaires can be used to assess both quantitative and qualitative factors.

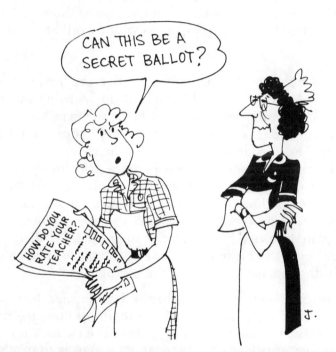

However, since the wording of the questionnaire may often determine the type of answer received, it would be advisable for the teacher-practitioner who wishes to evaluate by questionnaire to seek advice from others, e.g. researchers, psychologists or educationalists, as to its compilation. The validity of a questionnaire given to a learner or client after a one-to-one teaching encounter is open to question. Both client and student may feel they are in a vulnerable position which may cause bias in their answers. The student has to continue to gain experience and possibly be assessed by the qualified practitioner. The patient or client is part of a captive audience and so may lack confidence in speaking what he or she sees as the truth. In addition to these points, great care should be taken in the use of **closed** and **open** questions.

Bradshaw (1989) provides pointers for the novice on questionnaire formulation and is worth reading. The individual teacher may choose to design a questionnaire aimed solely at improving his or her own teaching style; this should be made clear to the client or learner so that no misunderstanding occurs.

5. EXAMINING THE PURPOSE OF EVALUATION

The type of questions that are asked within an evaluation will depend on who is doing the evaluation and its purpose. As differing purposes of evaluation have already been explored, the following sections will examine evaluation from the perspective of the evaluator. Hence the view of:

1. The learner—the learner who practises reflective thinking as a method of evaluation could find that the learning she has acquired during a teaching session, is not what she expected. In place of, or in addition to, the expected subject area there could be a hidden agenda. For example, the student may accompany a teacher-practitioner to observe her give advice prior to the discharge from hospital of a patient or client. It could emerge that whilst the teacher-practitioner is negotiating future support for the patient or client, she discovers unknown anxiety and problems. The learner will gain knowledge not just of planning for discharge for the patient/client but also knowledge of the skills of communication in which the teacher-practitioner has expertise.

2. The teacher—when the teacher is evaluating, does she consider merely what she believes she has taught, or does she find out what the student has learnt? It may be that the two are not the same. A teacher-practitioner may, for example, prepare to teach a student a skilled procedure such as applying suction to an endo-tracheal tube. On completion of this planned teaching session relatives, who have not previously seen the patient/client, may arrive to visit. The student may then learn the different skill of coping with anxious relatives. The student may gain far more from this learning encounter than was originally planned by the teacher-practitioner, and such unplanned learning should be accounted for on evaluation.

3. The outside perspective, i.e. Education Division or Health Authority: their criteria for evaluation are likely to be much wider and this aspect will be dealt with later in the chapter.

4. Jarvis and Gibson (1985) explore the value of 'peer' assessment or evaluation. Where two or more learners work together within a

clinical area, there is opportunity for the learners to observe one another and then discuss the points observed. Difficulties with this type of evaluation include unrealistic expectations of the learners and hidden or unknown relationships between the students. Any use of peer review will need careful and skilled guidance from the teacher-practitioner, who in turn ought to set clearly defined expected outcomes from the encounter.

6. WHEN SHOULD EVALUATION OCCUR?

Harris and Bell (1986) suggest that there are three parts to the evaluation process. Their first part has already been discussed in the initial sections of this chapter; you will recall they define preparatory evaluation as 'needs analysis', and this was discussed in relation to objectives, outcomes, SWOT analysis and standard setting. The other types of evaluation described by Harris and Bell are formative and summative. As there continues to be overlap and integration of the terms assessment and evaluation, it is useful here to take the two terms as synonymous and consider Jarvis and Gibson's (1985) definitions of the terms formative and summative which apply equally to both evaluation and assessment. Jarvis and Gibson also identified a third type of assessment as **continuous**. Their interpretation of the terms are as follows:

formative: diagnostic assessment, which occurs during the teaching and learning programme.

summative: a final assessment, which occurs at the end of a course such as an examination or an end-of-unit assignment.

continuing or **continuous**:   where assessment is regarded as an ongoing process through the course.

Narrow (1979), considering evaluation of teaching of patients, suggested that there are two main aspects: teaching effectiveness and teacher performance. She states that 'evaluation is the assessment of learning that has taken place.' One can argue that evaluation is ongoing and an integral part of reflection on any aspect of life, as you ask yourself, did I buy the right car? Was it the best value? Does it serve my purpose? The student can ask herself—did I get the information I needed? Did I ask suitable questions? The teacher may ask—did I give too little or too much information? Was it paced correctly? Did I give the student or client sufficient opportunity to question? What evidence have I got that learning has taken place?

Assessment of learning in clinical locations for the students of nursing and midwifery is most likely to be ongoing or continuous. Well-refined assessment processes usually include mid-point formative assessment, to give the learner an indication of their achievement to date or possible weaknesses. Methods of self-evaluation may also be included in the routine documentation. Any self-evaluation should be carried out by the learner prior to the teacher's assessment.

Midpoint formative assessment is less easy in the teaching situation with a client or patient than with a student of nursing or midwifery. However, the need for feedback and assessment of learning as an ongoing activity with patients/clients should not be minimised. In primary nursing, where goals are jointly set between client and practitioner, inbuilt assessment of learning can be planned. The evaluation phase of the nursing process should be seen as an ongoing process and not merely a summative phase. The person with learning difficulties will require continuous assessment and nursing goals will need to be evaluated on a regular basis as that person is helped to achieve their independent potential.

How do we decide the frequency of evaluation? Should it be ongoing or at the end of a given period of time? Narrow (1979) believes that it depends on the nature and amount of the material to be learned and on the time available to teach it. Another aspect to consider is 'when' should the evaluation take place in relation to the completion of a course? Summative evaluation will often present a different picture to evaluation carried out several months or more after completion of the course. Minor problems (e.g. with the environment in which learning takes place) may seem of lesser importance when there is opportunity for a realisation of the amount of learning that has taken place.

7. TRIANGULATION

Although Kenworthy and Nicklin (1989) discuss triangulation as a modified teacher-researcher model, for the purposes of the teacher-practitioner as an evaluator, triangulation will be considered separately. Triangulation is a method of evaluation where the learning encounter is viewed from several differing perspectives. Carry out the following activity in order to help you decide who should carry out the evaluation.

Activity 5.4.4.

Recall any teaching session in which you have taken part during the last week. Who do you think is in a position to evaluate the effectiveness of that teaching session?

Consider the student of nursing gaining experience with a Health

Visitor. The student is observing the Health Visitor carry out routine developmental screening on a six-week-old baby. During this developmental test the Health Visitor explains to both the student and the parent of the child important points. The Health Visitor, as a skilled practitioner, ensures that the parameters of normal are explained and explored and her manner is educative and reassuring to the patient.

The Health Visitor, the student of nursing and the parent will all be in a position to evaluate the effectiveness of the teaching. Other interested parties could be the College of Nursing and Midwifery from a curriculum perspective, and also the Health Authority, who will be concerned with the efficiency of the Health Visitor within her sphere of work.

Taking a similar scenario within the hospital setting, you should easily be able to identify comparable figures of qualified nurse or midwife, student of nursing or midwifery, patient/client. The College of Nursing and Midwifery and the Health Authority will remain interested parties. If three of more of these identifiable individuals all carry out their own evaluation of the same situation, each is likely to see it from a different perspective. The combined results from the separate evaluations can be termed evalution by triangulation.

In assessing whether a student has achieved the set outcomes for a period of training, triangulation can be useful, as the teacher-practitioner, the student and the course tutor can make and share their judgements. Burnard (1988) has written a very useful paper on student self-evaluation and much can be gained from seriously considering employing self-evaluation as an integral part of the learning process.

The emphasis within the evaluation models already described tends to be on objectivity. Whilst objective methods of evaluation such as examinations, assignments and questionnaires are useful to curriculum planners in measuring the number of student successes, clinicians often require more than quantifiable information. The teacher-practitioner in the clinical area is more likely to be involved in small group teaching, possibly patient/client education or teaching students whilst they are caring for patients/clients. Rapid feedback to the learner is of greater benefit than feedback which occurs sometime after the event. There is no reason why the teacher-practitioner should not organise an immediate evalaution of a teaching encounter.

8. ADVANTAGES OF SELF-EVALUATION (Burnard 1988)

1.   Self-evaluation provides a means of identifying personal progress, enabling the student to clarify what is still to be learned. The teacher can then consider how past learning can be integrated with present learning. This can be viewed as a process of incorporation or synthesis.

2. Gaps in learning can be identified, which in turn may lead to reviewing expected outcomes. Stopping to take stock of what has been learned gives the opportunity to reflect and reassess.

3. Inviting feedback from others can enhance our own self-awareness and is part of self-evaluation. Being willing to ask others for feedback can be equally useful to the teacher or the learner. Both may find some surprises in how they are seen by others, but with careful negotiation, beneficial changes can be made.

4. Self-evaluation also helps to develop autonomy in learning, which represents a move away from the student being dependent on others for evaluation of progress.

Self-evaluation is today being practised in general, further and higher education, and Project 2000 courses for the training and education of nurses are no exception. Nursing and midwifery education now aims to provide maximum opportunity for the student to develop more autonomy, both in the production of their written work and in areas of clinical practice. In relation to the patient/client similar changes in practice are occurring. As the practitioner acts as the patient's/client's advocate, the patient/client is actively encouraged to take on a decision-making role in relation to his or her own health.

9. METHODS OF SELF-EVALUATION

These can include questionnaires, as previously discussed. Self and peer-evaluation can be in response to specific questions or an exploration of feelings. Keeping a reflective journal may be useful in helping to move the focus away from the cognitive domain, as growth within the affective domain is assessed.

Activity 5.4.5.

Design an evaluation questionnaire which you can use following a future teaching session with learner, patient/client or relative.

Decide first if you wish the questionnaire to collect quantifiable information (facts which can be collated numerically), or qualitative information (that gained by asking open questions).

On completion of the questionnaire, discuss it with a colleague or group of fellow learners and ask yourselves:

continued on next page

continued

1. Are all the questions clear and unambiguous?

2. Are the questions logical in sequence?

3. Will the questions elicit the information required? Are the questions relevant?

4. Who will be asked to complete the questionnaire?

5. When will the questionnaire be completed?

These are only some of the questions you might like to ask. Discuss this with your colleagues and add any additional ones so that you can develop this tool for future use.

10. WHY EVALUATE AT ALL? WHO WANTS THE INFORMATION?

When considering the various possible definitions of the word 'evaluation', it is also a useful exercise to look at the purpose of evaluation. Is the purpose to help the student, or the teacher-practitioner, or does it have wider implications? Nicklin and Kenworthy (1989) suggest that accountability and cost-effectiveness are rapidly becoming prime factors in evaluation. Should the teacher-practitioner take these into account, or are they of no relevance to the clinical situation? If the teacher sees her prime role as helping the student, then her evaluation of teaching may focus solely on assessing what the student has learnt, and time and efficiency factors will not be considered. However, the changing ethos within the National Health Service is more likely to make it essential that clinicians as teachers consider efficiency and economy in all aspects of their work.

In providing quality care and teaching, it may be argued that the time taken with the elderly patient in discussing and explaining his bronchitis should not be measured and costed. In discussions with practitioners, when the focus is on teaching students, practitioners are unanimous in their view that this must not be at the expense of patients/clients, however, the teacher-practitioner must recognise his or her responsibility for educating the practitioner of the future. In many areas it may be necessary to evaluate a programme of teaching in order to justify future programmes. Teaching that occurs in a clinical area on an *ad hoc* basis is less likely to gain support and increased resources from management than that which can be seen to relate clearly and closely to improved performance and quality.

Reviewing all you have read on evaluation so far, you should now be able to develop your own evaluation questionnaire, and will be able to decide how you can put the resulting evaluation to maximum use. If your aim is solely to improve your own teaching, then the evaluation will just concern yourself and the person you teach; however, if your teaching is part of a curriculum, a unit of a curriculum or one of a sequence of teaching sessions to clients, patients, or relatives, there will need to be feedback from all involved. Those of you wishing to effect change on a larger scale, or as part of a quality assurance project, will need to circulate the information much more widely, and ensure your audience is in a position to act on the information. Nurse/midwife managers and general managers may be in a better position to effect change than yourselves.

CONCLUSION

There are many methods of evaluation and which you choose is dependent on several factors which hinge on answers to the following questions:

1. On what are the criteria for measuring evaluation based?

2. What is the purpose of the evaluation?

3. Who is going to carry out the evaluation?

4. Who needs the information gained?

Following definition and discussion of behavioural objectives, outcomes, performance indicators, standards, needs analysis and self-evaluation, you may have made your choice of the criteria you will use for evaluating your teaching. It does not matter if you have not yet made this choice, for as each teaching situation arises, one type of criterion may appear particularly pertinent in that situation. For example, if you are teaching a planned session and have the opportunity to negotiate with the learner prior to the teaching encounter, you may wish to consider needs analysis and planned outcomes for teaching. If a clinical area has set standards and/or performance indicators, then they may be adapted by you as you design your evaluation process.

Remember that the teaching method may be dictated by the subject being taught. Learning that is dependent on an attitude change will not require the same selection of teaching skills, for example, as learning that is behavioural and therefore measureable. The simplest way of measuring behaviour is by the use of behavioural objectives, detailing specific aspects of observable behaviour which can be checked against a criteria sheet of objectives. Discussion of feelings, and exploration of attitudes may be a more relevant method of evaluation to measure changes outside the behavioural domain. Sometimes the teaching method is dictated by the subject, for example, you would not be able to teach an aseptic dressing technique effectively without using special equipment and demonstrating your own skills. However, a topic that emphasises communication skills can be taught by a variety of methods and negotiation with learners regarding their preferred learning styles can be undertaken. The type of criteria for evaluation will therefore be dependent on the method of teaching used.

Sequentially, teaching methods ought to follow your setting of criteria, but there are usually exceptions to all general rules. You may have already decided that each teaching encounter requires a different kind of evaluation, and for each session you may methodically select the one you feel best fits the bill and with which you are at ease.

You have been urged to consider whether the purpose of evaluation is to improve your own teaching, or improve learning, and should the learning environment be considered? The answers you give to these questions will provide you with clues to who should carry out the evaluation. If you personally are responsible for the learning climate, then it will be up to you to carry out the evaluation and take appropriate action. The diversity of thought and choices of evaluation strategies should not deter you from including evaluation as part of your practice as a teacher-practitioner. With rapid changes in the ethos and philosophy of practice, evaluation is more important than ever. We are only able to progress, move forward, if knowledgeable practitioners not only question, but take action on the answers they receive. Evaluation is an important, exciting part of the teaching-learning process and the skilled teacher-practitioner will integrate it into practice with enjoyment.

GLOSSARY

Closed questions: these expect a relatively set answer, and do not normally give opportunity for expansion, or more than a few words, e.g. What is your name? Do you want a bath? Have you any pain?

Continuing or continuous assessment: where assessment is regarded as an ongoing process throughout the course.

Experiential learning: learning that has occurred as a result of a combination of 'learning through doing' and planned teaching, which may or not incorporate 'role play', but which does include open discussion and sharing of experiences and feelings.

Formative assessment: diagnostic assessment which occurs during the teaching and learning programme.

Open questions: give the opportunity for expansive answers and elicit more information, e.g. How do you feel today? What would you like to learn about child care this afternoon?

Outcomes: refers to the resulting change in knowledge, attitude or skill following a teaching/learning encounter.

Qualitative: information which gives some indication of the quality of what has taken place but to which a numerical value is not or cannot be assigned.

Quantitative: information which can be analysed to produce measurable facts and figures.

Summative assessment: a final assessment that occurs at the end of a course such as an examination or an end-of-unit assignment.

REFERENCES

Andrusyszyn M A (1989) Clinical Evaluation of the Affective Domain. *Nurse Education Today*, **9**, 75–81.

Armitage P and Burnard P (1991) Mentors or Preceptors? Narrowing the theory–practice gap. *Nurse Education Today*, **11**, 225–229.

Balogh R, Beattie A and Beckerleg S (1989) *Figuring out Performance*. London: English National Board for Nursing Midwifery and Health Visiting.

Benner P (1984) *From Novice to Expert*. California: Addison Wesley.

Bloom B S, Madaus G F and Hastings J T (1981) *Evaluation to Improve Learning*. London: McGraw-Hill.

Bradshaw P L (1989) *Teaching and Assessing in Clinical Nursing Practice*. London: Prentice Hall.

Burnard P (1988) Self-evaluation Methods in Nurse Education. *Nurse Education Today*, **8**, 229–223.

Burnard P (1990) The Student Experience: adult learning and mentorship revisited. *Nurse Education Today*, **10**, 349–354.

Department of Health (1989) Project 2000. A Guide to Implementation Documentation from the Department of Health Project 2000 implementation group, released through Regional Health Authorities to Districts submitting bids for April 1990 start dates. North West Regional Health Authority covering letter dated 13th Oct 1990. Supported by EL(89) P/191 and EL(90) P/25 Department of Health Advance Letters.

Donabedian A (1966) Evaluating the Quality of Medical Care. *Milbank Memorial Fund Quarterly*, XLI, 3(2), 166–205.

Fretwell J (1982) *Ward Teaching and Learning: Sister and the Learning Environment*. London: Royal College of Nursing.

Fretwell J (1985) *Freedom to Change: The Creation of a Ward Learning Environment*. London: Royal College of Nursing.

Harris D and Bell C (1986) *Evaluating and Assessing for Learning*. London: Kogan Page.

Hinchliff S (1986) *Teaching Clinical Nursing* (2nd edn). Edinburgh: Churchill Livingstone.

Jarvis P and Gibson S (1985) *The Teacher Practitioner in Nursing Midwifery and Health Visiting*. London: Croom Helm.

Kenworthy N and Nicklin P (1989) *Teaching and Assessing in Nursing Practice*. London: Scutari Press.

Kitson A, Hyndman S, Harvey G and Yerrell P (1990) *Quality Patient Care, the Dynamic Standard Setting System*. Royal College of Nursing. London: Scutari Press.

Kotler P (1988) *Marketing Management: Analysis, Planning, Implementation and Control* (6th edn). London: Prentice-Hall.

Lawton D (1983) *Curriculum Studies and Educational Planning*. London: Hodder and Stoughton.

Litwack L L (1979) Meeting the Challenge of Clinical Evaluation. National League for Nursing: the challenge of clinical evaluation, Pub. No. 16, p. 1763 New York: NLN 1–15, cited in Andrusyszyn, M A (1989) Clinical evaluation of the affective domain, *Nurse Education Today*, **9**, 75–81.

Mager R F (1984) *Goal Analysis* (2nd edn). London: Pitman Press.

Marson S (1987) Learning for Change: developing the 'teaching' role of the ward sister. *Nurse Education Today*, **7**, 103–108.

Mogan J and Knox J E (1987) Characteristics of 'Best' and 'Worst' Clinical Teachers as Perceived by University Nursing Faculty and Students. *Journal of Advanced Nursing*, **12**, 331–337.

Narrow B W (1979) *Patient Teaching in Nursing Practice*. John Wiley and Sons, USA.

Ogier M (1982) *An Ideal Sister? A Study of the Leadership Style and Verbal Interactions of Ward Sisters with Nurse Learners in General Hospitals*. London: Royal College of Nursing.

Orton H (1981) *Ward Learning Climate*. London: Royal College of Nursing.

The Report of the Post-Registration Education and Practice Project (1990) London: United Kingdom Central Council for Nursing Midwifery and Health Visiting.

Reid N G (1985) *Wards in Chancery—nurse training in the clinical area*. London: Royal College of Nursing.

Spouse J (1990) *An Ethos for Learning*. London: Scutari Press.

Wheeler D (1970) *Curriculum Process*. London University, London Press.

FURTHER READING

Andrusyszyn M A (1989) Clinical Evaluation of the Affective Domain, *Nurse Education Today*, **9**, 75–81. This paper considers the strengths and limitations of evaluating in the affective domain. It has a useful, easy to follow style which deals with a subject area which some find difficult to explore. Suggestions for methods of evaluating the affective domain are included.

Kitson A, Hyndman S, Harvey G and Yerrell P (1990) *Quality Patient Care, the Dynamic Standard Setting System.* Royal College of Nursing. London: Scutari Press. This slim workbook is designed specifically as a teaching pack. The text is set out clearly and the reader is given the opportunity to work at his/her own pace in developing an understanding of Standard Setting and Quality Patient Care.

Spouse J (1990) *An Ethos for Learning.* London: Scutari Press. This research report begins with a very useful literature review on learning environments. Previous research reports on this subject are thoroughly discussed, and their findings built upon for Spouse's own investigation. Results are clearly set out and provide a sound basis for any practitioner-teacher improving his or her clinical learning environment.

Chapter 6
Applying Teaching Skills in Practice

This concluding chapter will focus on teaching in the clinical area. First though, we will present a brief overview of theories and models and consider how these are related to the delivery of care, using a problem-solving approach. This problem-solving approach or systematic approach to care is not, in itself, a model/framework for practice but rather a means of implementation. There are those who claim that models of care arose from clinical practice by analysing what nursing is about and how it is delivered: for example, Roy (1984) and Orem (1985). Others such as Rogers (1970) and King (1981) suggest that the theoretical framework was developed first and that the guidelines for practice evolved from this. The intention of this section is not to argue for or against either view, but for you to explore how care is delivered in your area and how you can enable those who come to you for experience to learn about approaches to care. It may be that you are working towards the implementation of a model of nursing or midwifery care; if so, issues surrounding the introduction of any change are essential inclusions in your teaching strategy.

Florence Nightingale (1859) put forward what we would recognise as the earliest model of nursing. She identified those aspects of care she felt were important in caring for the sick. Since this time the concept of a 'model' for practice has diversified and evolved (Kershaw and Salvage 1986, Aggleton and Chalmers 1986, Riehl and Roy 1980).

6.1. EXAMINING YOUR AREA OF PRACTICE

Activity 6.1a.

Take some time at this point to revise your knowledge of the model

continued on next page

---

continued _____

> of care in use in your area of practice. Go to your College of Nursing or Midwifery library and read a synopsis of the model, first of all in one of the texts suggested above (these are termed *secondary sources*). Having done that consult the *primary source*, i.e. the writings of the model's originator. You will find clear references to these in the secondary sources cited above.

Each model contains certain common aspects. The terminology may vary slightly between American and British approaches, but basically the aspects can be described in the following terms:

1. The goal of care

2. a description of who the client/patient is

3. the role the practitioner plays in the implementation process

4. the problem or difficulty as perceived by the client/patient

5. the focus of the intervention

6. the mode of intervention

7. the desired outcomes.

Activity 6.1b.

Take each one of the above in turn and examine how they relate to the model you are using in your clinical area as a framework for practice.

Having familiarised yourself with the model of care used in your particular area, you need now to take time to consider the most appropriate method to adopt in order to teach patients/clients, student nurses or midwives or any one of a range of health care personnel about it.

> ## Activity 6.1c.
>
> Think back to chapter 3 where we discussed how to identify what to teach (section 3.2.3.(i)) and start to ask yourself what your colleagues need to know in order to use the framework effectively and what skills they need in order to put this knowledge into practice.

You may find it helpful to use Wright's (1990) fields of nursing knowledge to help you to identify what you need to teach. Wright suggested that nursing knowledge can be divided into a number of fields, as follows:

1. Nursing
What does nursing entail in your area of care? Are there any special skills that staff need? You need to be familiar with current research and how the framework chosen in your area affects the role of the practitioner.

2. Managing care
This relates to the way in which care is organised and delivered in your area and how involved the practitioners and students are in this, for example, do you use primary nursing or team midwifery?

3. Psychology/Social psychology
You will need to determine the 'role' of both the practitioner and the client/patient and how the environment affects both the individual and the group.

4. Sociological concepts
Here you might like to explore the value/belief systems of the practitioners and client/patient; the role of the care-giving environment; the sick role, disability and inequalities in care.

5. Illness
What do staff need to know about the patterns of illness related to your area, how to recognise the features of illness and its effects on self-care?

6. Related science/fields of study
This includes pharmacology, microbiology as associated with the role and function of the practitioner, for example in preventing cross-infection, nutrition and pathology.

7. Basic helping concepts

You will need to facilitate an understanding of the complexity of humans, dependence and independence, together with ways of developing skills in communications, relationships and stress reduction.

8. Homeostasis

Represents exploration of what the practitioner and student need to know about normal and disordered physiological functioning, pertinent to your area of practice.

Activity 6.1d.

Under these headings which we have identified for you, write down what you consider to be important subheadings.

To help you get started we are offering you some ideas. Add your ideas to our suggestions in the spaces provided. Remember that these are not listed in priority order.

Nursing

Under this heading you will need to explore:

philosophy   What is the approach to care in your area of practice?

 (i)   Is it individualised?

 (ii)   Does it include a description of the model/framework in use?

(iii)   Do you adopt a problem-solving approach to care?

You may wish to consider, under this subheading, the role of the patient/client in the care process.

practical skills   What do the staff need to be able to do in terms of practical skills in order to provide the care required? For instance, are there any specialised techniques they need to learn? What standards have been set?

professional development   Here you need to consider what you can offer practitioners in terms of professional development. You will need to emphasise the importance of continuing education in relation to your specialty and be familiar with what is available (you may wish to consult the educational manager responsible for continuing education at your college to help you with this).

nursing research   What research has been undertaken relating to your area of practice or what is being undertaken in your area? You may wish to visit your college library and obtain references to which you can direct staff. You could, of course, decide to compile your own resource packs for use in your area.

Managing Care
decision-making process   How involved are the staff in this? You will need to consider how decisions are made and describe the stages in the process

methods of organising care, e.g.   task allocation
team nursing
primary nursing

Why did your area decide on a particular approach to care and how is it put into practice? You may need to take time to explain the benefits to the client/patient and the role of the practitioner within the chosen approach.

learning climate of the clinical area   What is available for the staff in terms of experience and how is this organised to ensure maximal participation and achievement of learning outcomes? What are professional relationships like in your area? Is the ward/unit/area welcoming to learners, and accepting of the challenges they may present? Is a questioning/critical attitude fostered?

prevailing management style   You need to examine this very carefully and be very honest with yourself. Are team members' contributions taken into account and acted upon? How involved are both students and practitioners in the determination of priorities? What do you do in times of discontent or possible conflict? What support mechanisms are available? Can staff be sure of fair and confidential treatment (where appropriate)?

Psychology/Social Psychology
man and his environment   Who is the client/patient in relation to the practitioner? Are they equal partners in care? How does the environment affect recovery and what do you do to enhance this? How are relatives welcomed and treated?

developmental psychology   leads you to consider what is important for the practitioner or student to understand about the development of individuals and how knowing the client/patient as an individual within their own context can help the practitioner to determine the best approach to care.

Sociological Concepts

nurse–patient/client interaction   What is expected of the practitioner or the student? What does the practitioner say when faced with questions they do not really know how to answer? How much information do they feel able to give? Have clients access to their personal records?

the sick role   What is the role of the client whilst in your area of practice? To what extent is the client/patient perceived as an individual? Are all clients required to wear night attire all day long? Think about the organisation of the client/patient day.

concepts of professionalism   What does it mean to be a professional practitioner? You may wish to discuss the code of professional conduct and how this relates to your particular area. You may wish to identify the various roles required of the practitioner, for example, counsellor, teacher, mentor, assessor.

Illness

— social patterns of disease

— epidemiology

— effects of illness on self-care

— clinical features

All of these are related to your own area of practice, for example, what are the commonly presenting client/patient problems? Are they more common in the part of the world in which you reside, or are they fairly common worldwide?

Related Science/Fields of Study

What other disciplines underpin practice in your clinical area?

To what extent is a knowledge of each of importance in assessing, planning, delivering, evaluating care?

Who is best placed to teach this?

What resources might be needed?

Basic Helping Concepts

adaptation   What is the practitioner's role in helping the client/patient to adapt to his current and future situation or possible disability? How do you set about establishing a relationship based on trust? What do the staff need to know about organisations available to the client/patient following discharge? What coping mechanisms might clients use?

culture   An awareness of the dangers of stereotyping clients/patients is important, as is an awareness of the background of the client/patient in relation to ethnic origins and religious beliefs, etc.

threat   Practitioners need help in recognising situations which instill fear or anxiety in patients/clients and the appropriate action to take in order to avoid them (for example pain, and the defence mechanisms the client may adopt).

Homeostasis
— structure and function of the body

— interdependent nature of bodily functions

— nutrition

— fluid and electrolyte balance

The above should be related to your own area of practice. What do students or practitioners new to your area need to know about the above in relation to your client/patient group?

These are just a few of the many facets of nursing knowledge required. Perhaps you can use these to build on, involving members of your care team, to put together a comprehensive list for your clinical area. Alternatively, you may decide to compile a different list using your own headings.

How then do you set about making sure that you cover all the necessary information, so that staff have the opportunity to maximise their learning? You might decide to develop a scheme of work, so you and your clinical colleagues have a clear picture of what is required.

6.2. PREPARING A SCHEME OF WORK

As you read this section, and especially if you undertake this exercise, refer back frequently to the relevant sections in chapter 3, *Planning for Teaching*.

Consider first of all what you need to:

1. *Know*

Week No.	Topic	Competency	Teaching method	Learning resources	Time allowed	Assessment of Learning	Responsible for the Session
1 DAY ONE	Orientation to the clinical area and discussion of learning opportunities. Discussion regarding competencies to be achieved and methods of assessment. Introduction to staff.	B. Recognise situations that may be detrimental to the health and well being of the individual. A. Advise on the promotion of health and prevention of illness	Discussion Explanation Show round the ward — fire escapes — fire equipment — patient notes — resuscitation equipment — handbook for patient/staff working with staff	Staff handbooks Handouts Wallcharts Scheme of work Student's assessment record Policy documents	All day at intervals when appropriate. Initial orientation 1½ hrs.	Question and answer direct observation	Initially Sister/Deputy. Then delegated staff member. Primarily the student's mentor.
1	Philosophy of care	A.	Explanation of issues underpinning philosophy — Assess student's level of knowledge	Handbook diagram of how philosophy relates to care — articles — textbooks	Wed pm 3–4 / Thurs Over lunch 12.30–1.15	Check understanding — questions & answers — student's recap	Sister/Staff Nurse
1	The model/framework	C. Carry out those activities involved when conducting the comprehensive assessment of a person's nursing requirements.	Assess level of understanding — explain as required — explanation of documentation — how to take a nursing history	— Nursing histories outline handout of main points. — Articles of interest — staff	1 hour / As long as required over the period of the shift	Check understanding clarification / Student to take nursing history under supervision — completion of relevant documentation — reflect on activity — feedback to student	Sister / Mentor/supervisor

AND SO ON

Figure 6.1. Outline of scheme of work (see also appendix 1)

- curriculum/course details for all your students
- stage of programme s/he is at
- previous knowledge pertaining to your area of practice
- method by which competence is to be assessed

Next you need to:

2. *Decide*

   - what the student   *must*
                              should
                              could learn, in order to achieve the
                                       competencies.

3.   Then you need to *consider the educational principles* involved in teaching the topics. In particular the need:

- for a holistic approach
- to move from the known to the unknown, when teaching
- to move from simple to complex
- to divide the content to be learned into manageable portions, perhaps in weeks
- to prepare learning outcomes

4.   Finally consider:

- the *appropriate method* of teaching/learning for each session
- what *learning resources* are needed and what are available
- the *time allowed* for each session
- *how learning will be assessed.*

5.   Produce *detailed references* and *further reading* material.

This is a very brief outline to which you can add your own ideas. It is important that everyone involved is familiar with the scheme of work, so it should be displayed in a prominent place in the clinical area. Figure 6.1 suggests a layout for a scheme of work which you could adapt to suit your own needs and those of your care-team. (See appendix 1 for brief outlines of competences A–I.)

Having identified what you need to include in your scheme of work and the timescale involved, you need to consider the sequencing of events, that is, what staff new to your clinical area need to know first. If a particular framework for practice is used, then it is likely that in the preparation period, prior to the student attending the clinical area for experience, s/he will have had sessions in the College of Nursing/Midwifery related to models/frameworks for practice.

Activity 6.2a.

Contact the teachers responsible for Pre/Post-registration courses (as appropriate) and discuss exactly what students have been taught before they come to your area on placement. It is possible that you may be able to 'sit in' on some of the sessions.

Once you know what the student has undertaken by way of preparation you can use this information to assess what the student has learned, so that you have a baseline on which to build, in terms of applying the theory to practice.

Activity 6.2b.

Refer back now to chapter 3 on *Planning for Teaching*. Using the material there on teaching methods, reflect on how best you can ensure the student gets optimal opportunities for learning.

The likelihood is you will choose to adopt a range of activities and methods relevant to the learning situation. For example, there will be times when it is appropriate to:

- discuss/explain the reasoning behind decisions/activities
- provide opportunities for experiential learning, for example, encour-

aging students to take a history (under supervision) and giving appropriate feedback to increase the student's confidence.

- encouraging the student to become more reflective about the process of care delivery both whilst delivering it and afterwards.

Activity 6.2c.

Refer back to chapters 1 and 2 and refresh your memory of experiential learning, then refer to the section related to experiential learning in chapter 3. Take some time over this and see if you can design your own session, based on this approach. Use a simple example and see how it works. From this you can move on to more complex situations. By this stage, you have all the information required to carry out this exercise, but if it proves too difficult, go and see one of the teachers in the college and ask for their advice and guidance.

Whilst each theorist shares some common themes, there are obvious differences in the way caring is perceived. However, each model/framework stresses and defines the role of the practitioner. The uniqueness of the model/framework stems from the way in which the practitioner intervenes.

Activity 6.2d.

Consider the key elements of the practitioner's role in your chosen model/framework.

This will give you some indication of the skills required and so will help you plan what to teach. For instance, you need to ascertain whether the role is concerned with being:

- insightful

- a counsellor

- a change agent

- assisting the patient/client to make any adaptive changes necessary.

It is important for you at all times to remember the level (or readiness) of the student you are teaching, and what is appropriate for that student to know and be able to do. This is emphasised in chapter 1 (1.7c).

Activity 6.2e.

Having familiarised yourself with the experiential learning cycle, refer back to chapter 1, Fig. 1.3, The reflective learning cycle.

Consider your own area of clinical practice and the type of experience the student may encounter. Select one experience with which you are confident and feel comfortable exploring with the student or client/patient.

How would you employ this technique?

If you recall from chapter 1, the reflective cycle has three stages:

1. the experience

2. the reflective process

3. the outcomes

Firstly, consider your approach to a student.

Stage 1
The student is asked to recall the experience and highlight the important points.

How could you initiate and develop this?

You may find it worthwhile to practise this on your own, so that you have a chance to consider what the student may come up with.

You could, of course, reflect on your own earlier experience in similar situations.

Stage 2
Requires you and the student to focus on the student's feelings about the experience, including both positive and negative aspects.

How will you prepare yourself for this?

You may consider sharing your own experiences with the student.

Stage 3
Involves re-evaluating the experience in the light of reflection. Perhaps you may wish, at this point, to highlight the strengths the student has exhibited throughout the experience and together with the student develop an action plan to overcome the areas which the student identified as needing further development.

Activity 6.2f.

You may wish to consider undertaking a similar exercise with a client/patient. To help you to plan this there is a very good example contained in the section 'Teaching through the reflective process' in chapter 1. Read the example about the client in a self-propelled wheelchair. Can you think of a situation in your own area of practice where you could employ a similar strategy?

Miles (1987) gives a description of how you can use the student's experience and build on it to maximise learning in the clinical area.

Activity 6.2g.

In chapter 1, there is an example in the section entitled 'Teaching from a student's experience', which is based on the work of Benner (*From Novice to Expert*, 1984).

Using this example, try to develop your own approach by substituting a situation with which you are familiar.

Boud et al (1985) describe the process of developing a learning experience by using a reflective cycle (see chapter 1, Figure 1.3). Schön (1987) advocates the usefulness of reflective processes in helping others to make decisions under conditions of uncertainty, by:

1.   thinking back on the action:
What was positive and what was negative?
What did the individual do that they would not do now?
Have they learned from their mistakes?
What was the client/patient reaction?

2.   stopping and thinking, either before or in mid-action:
Is the approach the right approach?
Is what you are doing likely to cause distress? If so, how can you minimise this?
Are you sure about what you are doing?

You might like to include here any other points which you feel are appropriate to consider.

Activity 6.2h.

What methods can you think of which you could use to develop reflective practice? How would you implement these?

It is important to remember that whatever you decide to implement in relation to teaching and learning, the student will at all times need appropriate guidance. Learning which begins with the experience and is followed by reflection, analysis and evaluation is described by Wright, 1970 (see chapter 2 for details).

You may find it useful to refer to chapter 3 *Planning for teaching* to help you with this.

CONCLUSION

By working through this book you have had the opportunity to examine, explore and expand your knowledge of:

• the nature of teaching and learning

- assessing learning needs

- planning for teaching

- the process of teaching

- evaluating your effectiveness as a teacher.

You have been actively involved in your own learning and the determination of your own level of achievement and you should now feel much more confident in your role as a teacher-practitioner. It is not expected that you will remember everything you have covered in working through this book—but you have a very valuable resource for reference purposes.

Enjoy your newly acquired skills and knowledge—your students certainly will.

REFERENCES

Aggleton P and Chalmers H (1986) *Nursing Models and the Nursing Process.* London: Macmillan.

Benner P (1984) *From Novice to Expert.* California: Addison Wesley.

Boud D, Keogh R and Walker D (1985) *Reflections: Training Experience into learning.* London: Kogan Page.

Kershaw B and Salvage J (1986) *Models for Nursing.* London: Wiley.

King I M (1981) *A Theory of Nursing: systems concepts process* New York: Wiley.

Miles R (1987) Experiential learning in the curriculum, in Allan P and Jolley M *The Curriculum in Nurse Education.* London: Croom Helm.

Nightingale F (1859) *Notes on Nursing* (New edition 1970). London: Duckworth.

Orem D (1985) *Nursing: Concepts of Practice* (3rd edn). New York: McGraw-Hill.

Riehl J P and Roy C (Eds) (1980) *Conceptual Models for Nursing Practice.* Norwalk CT: Appleton-Century-Crofts.

Rogers M (1970) *An Introduction to the Theoretical Basis for Nursing.* Philadelphia: Davis.

Roy C (1984) *Introduction to Nursing: An Adaptation Model* (3rd edn). New Jersey: Prentice Hall.

Schon D A (1987) *Educating the Reflective Practitioner.* London: Jossey Bass.

Wright D (1970) *Handbook for the Assessment of Experiential Learning from Experience Trust.* London: Twentieth Century Press.

Wright S G (1990) *Building and Using a Model of Nursing* (2nd edn) London: Edward Arnold.

FURTHER READING

Parse R (1987) *Nursing Science: Major Paradigms, Theories and Critiques.* Philadelphia: Harcourt, Brace Jovanovich. This book is worth using as a resource. It critiques the following: Roy's adaptation model, Orem's theory,

King's theory, Roger's framework. This is a fairly detailed book, which requires concentration; it does contain very useful information.

Fitzpatrick J and Whall A (1983) *Conceptual Models of Nursing: Analysis and Application*. New Jersey: Prentice Hall. This is a comprehensive text which explores a number of models/frameworks, including Nightingale's visionary model for nursing. It also contains a useful comparison chart of the models discussed. It is a fairly straightforward book, but you may find some of the terminology slightly complicated.

There are many other books of this nature, so visit your own college library and browse, until you find the book which answers your questions in the way you understand.

APPENDIX 1

The following pages contain a brief outline of the way in which you may assess competencies A–I as expressed in The Nurses, Midwives and Health Visitors Rules Approval Order, 1983.

They are by no means the only methods, but may serve to direct your thoughts.

You will note that for each competency the ways in which it can be assessed are divided into the cognitive, psychomotor and affective domains.

Advise on the promotion of health and prevention of illness (Competency a)

Cognitive
1. Demonstrate knowledge of different socio-cultural, economic and environmental factors, and their effects upon the individual's health and well-being.

2. Demonstrate an understanding of altered physiological states.

3. Make available to the patients the appropriate persons/resources to prevent stress affecting the physiological, psychological and social well-being of the individual.

4. Describe the role of the nurse in relation to Health Education.

5. Identify the needs of an individual to attain and maintain health and well-being.

Psychomotor
1. Apply necessary factors to improve general health and well-being of all patients in his/her charge.

2. Recognise and apply appropriate principles when dealing with patients experiencing a difference in their normal health states.

3. Make available to the patients the appropriate persons/resources to prevent stress affecting the physiological, psychological and social well-being of the individual.

4. Participate in and promote teaching of Health Education and its importance in relation to a healthy life.

5. Organise and carry out those activities which will promote health and well-being of the individual, applying research findings where applicable.

Affective

1. Show the need to maintain dignity, individuality and independence for all patients.

2. Appreciate the difference between normal and abnormal states of health.

3. (a) Show sensitivity towards the emotional and socio-economic aspects of patients and their relatives.
   (b) Explain the value of reducing the effects of those factors that create a stressful environment.

4. Recognise and appreciate the need for a multidisciplinary team.

5. (a) Display tact and diplomacy when dealing with the individual and their relatives.
   (b) Identify the necessity for a balance between the freedom of the individual and his needs and capabilities, when advising about promotion of health and well-being.

Recognise situations that may be detrimental to the health and well-being of the individual (Competency b)

Cognitive

1. Recognise situations in the environment (both ward and general areas) that can be potentially hazardous to the individual.

2. Explain the Health Authority's policies, e.g. fire, drug policies.

3. Explain and compare the correct techniques for lifting and moving patients. Describe the use of aids, according to manufacturers' instructions.

4. Relate knowledge of pathogenic organisms to the mode of spread and prevention and control of infection and infestation.

5. Explain the need to communicate effectively.

Psychomotor
1. (a) Display an ability to prevent hazardous situations arising for the individual.
   (b) Organise a safe and quiet environment for each patient and report and record correctly any accident or incident.
2. Implement the Health Authority's policies, as and when required.
3. Plan and demonstrate the correct lifting and moving of patients and use of equipment.
4. Demonstrate the ability to practise and relate this knowledge to the ward and general areas.
5. Display the appropriate verbal/written methods of communication to maintain individuals' safety.

Affective
1. Propose measures to prevent hazardous situations which could be detrimental to the well-being of the individual.
2. Recognise the need to adhere to local and national policies with regard to health and safety and legality of care.
3. Appreciate safety consciousness relating to lifting and moving patients and be fully aware of the risks and legal implications of using wrong methods.
4. Recognise the importance and accept the responsibility for the prevention of cross-infection and the need for education in these areas.
5. Recognise the need for effective communication in all forms.

Carry out those activities involved when conducting the comprehensive assessment of a person's nursing requirements (Competency c)

Cognitive
1. Recognise and display the knowledge required to complete a comprehensive nursing history, which should be accurate, confidential and legally compliable.

2. Demonstrate the importance of relating a model of nursing to display an holistic view.

3. Critically review the image/values/beliefs of self.

4.   Analyse the individual's personal reaction towards the assessment, realising the patient's own perceptions of his situation, his needs and his problems.

5.   Recognise the complexity of the requirements needed for effective interviewing and assessment of an individual.

Psychomotor

1.   Select and conduct the physical, psychological, social and spiritual assessment of the individual.

2.   Select and apply the appropriate nursing model.

3.   Demonstrate skill in being non-judgemental of others' values, beliefs and opinions.

4.   Encourage the individual's participation in the assessment of his needs and problems.

5.   Demonstrate effective communication skills within the patient/client, practitioner/relative, practitioner/practitioner, practitioner/doctor relationship.

Affective

1.   Appreciate that accuracy, confidentiality and legal compliance are essential in compiling data, and adopt the appropriate manner to achieve this.

2.   Appreciate the use of selective individualised care as displayed in an holistic approach.

3.   Respect the values, beliefs and opinions of others.

4.   Recognise the unique position of the individual and his or her sensitivity towards interpersonal behaviours.

5.   Appreciate the emotional, psychological and physical effects a situation may provoke in an individual.

Recognise the significance of the observations made and use these to develop an initial nursing assessment (Competency d)

Cognitive

1.   Recognise what is meant by the problem-solving approach and identify its place within the overall concept of a nursing model.

2.   Identify the many areas of assessment required, and the limitations of more junior nurses in perceiving them.

3.   Recognise the effect on the individual of common pathological and traumatic conditions. Relate these physiological changes to the needs of the individual.

Psychomotor

1.   Demonstrate skill in choosing the appropriate nursing model of care.

2.   Direct and facilitate the learning of other nurses, using all available resources.

3.   Demonstrate the skill of relating the observations made to the physiological, physical, social and psychological activities of the individual.

Affective

1.   Appreciate the problem-solving approach, formulating a correct concept of the appropriate nursing model.

2.   Display positive encouragement and empathy to the education of other nurses.

3.   Accept the link between the environment and the observations made of the individual.

Devise a plan of nursing care based on the assessment with the co-operation of a patient (to the extent that this is possible) taking into account the medical prescription (Competency e)

Cognitive

1.   Identify the various nursing models and justify the use of a particular model when devising a nursing care-plan.

2.   (a) Justify the reasons for negotiating the care plan with the individual/relatives and the care team.
     (b) Select the methods used to gain the trust and confidence of the individual/relatives.

3.   Demonstrate knowledge and skill in teaching others the relevant aspects of nursing care.

4.   Identify the accountability and responsibility of the nurse with regard to compiling care plans, concerning the ethical and legal implications.

Psychomotor
1.   Devise a plan of nursing care using a model of nursing.

2.   (a) Negotiate and communicate the care plan with the individual/
     relatives and the care team.
     (b) Begin organising a trustworthy environment when dealing with
     the individual and his relatives.

3.   Facilitate the caring process and promote the benefits of indivi-
     dualised care within a concept of a nursing model.

4.   Display legibility, conciseness, and ethical and legal correctness in
     all aspects of practice.

Affective
1.   Critically look at and evaluate the chosen nursing model.

2.   Display the following characteristics of a nurse:
     —loyalty to the individual and his relatives,
     —respect for belief, culture and values,
     —honesty and empathy,
     —receptivity to ideas,
     —approachability, enabling the individual/relatives and others to
     voice their opinions.

3.   Show sensitivity in creating an atmosphere conducive to teaching
     and learning interpersonal skills and their relevant application to
     nursing care.

4.   Appreciate the need for devising and maintaining accurate plans of
     nursing care.

**Implement the planned programme of nursing care and, where
appropriate, teach and co-ordinate other members of the caring
team who may be responsible for implementing specific aspects
of the nursing care (Competency f)**

Cognitive
1.   Identify the nursing care needs of individuals in your charge, using
     a nursing model.

2.   Demonstrate correct use of concepts and principles of safe adminis-
     tration of medicines.

3.   Identify the needs, in preparation for investigations/procedures,
     required by individuals.

4. Understand the need for policies/procedures as stated and laid down by the Health Authority.

5. Identify factors which constitute an emergency situation.

Psychomotor
1. (a) Create an environment in which privacy, dignity and individuality can be provided.
    (b) Set a high standard of nursing care, by example, through your own practice.

2. Demonstrate skill in safely carrying out administration of all medicines.

3. (a) Prepare individuals and provide continued care.
    (b) Demonstrate to student nurses, through your own practice, appropriate understanding and adaptation in caring for individuals.

4. Execute practice in a professional manner and act as a role model at all times.

5. Implement emergency care when required and efficiently assist other disciplines in these situations.

Affective
1. (a) Accept your own responsibility for providing/delegating nursing care according to the needs of the individual.
    (b) Motivate all members of the caring team to provide individual care.

2. Accept responsibility for safe administration of medicines.

3. Show appropriate understanding and adaptation whilst providing the emotional and psychological support identified, as required by individuals.

4. Appreciate legal and professional responsibility.

5. Show the appropriate urgency when dealing with emergency situations.

Review the effectiveness of the nursing care provided and when appropriate, initiate any action that may be required (Competency g)

Cognitive
   1.   Identify the appropriate methods needed to evaluate the effective-
        ness of the nursing care provided for the individual.

   2.   Recognise the sources for obtaining information regarding the effec-
        tiveness of care provided.

   3.   Critically judge the validity and effectiveness of information
        received.

Psychomotor
   1.   (a) Evaluate the changing needs of the individual.
        (b) Where appropriate, initiate plans to meet the changing needs of
            the individual.
        (c) Confirm, by assisting student nurses, the practicality of the
            nursing prescription (plan).

   2.   Demonstrate verbal and written skills in passing on information
        regarding effectiveness of nursing care.

   3.   Produce legible, concise and legally acceptable documentation.

Affective
   1.   (a) Appreciate the need to evaluate care prescribed, frequently and
            use different methods of evaluation.
        (b) Appreciate the importance of confidentiality and the rights of
            the patient.
        (c) Accept the need to involve the individual and others in chang-
            ing the care provided.

   2.   Accept responsibility for accurately recording and reporting on the
        effectiveness of nursing care.

   3.   Accept responsibility for accurately recording and reporting data
        received.

Work in a team with other nurses and with medical/para-medical staff and social workers (Competency h)

Cognitive
   1.   Identify the roles of other members of the caring team in relation to
        the needs of individuals.

   2.   Recognise one's own limitations.

   3.   Recognise the importance of maintaining effective communications
        and good relations within the caring team.

Psychomotor
1. Demonstrate skills in co-ordination of members of the caring team.

2. (a) Utilise appropriate personnel to develop and improve performance.
   (b) Interact constructively with other members in maximising patient care.

3. (a) Utilise appropriate methods of communication effectively.
   (b) Demonstrate skill in personal and professional aptitude when interacting with other members of the caring team.

Affective
1. (a) Accept the necessity for inclusion of other members of the caring team.
   (b) Appreciate the usefulness of skills of other members of the caring team.

2. Accept one's own limitations.

3. Accept the need to be:
   — reliable
   — receptive to the needs of others
   — receptive to advice and guidance.

Undertake the management of the care of a group of patients over a period of time and organise appropriate support services (Competency i)

Cognitive
1. State the role of the practitioner and outline her own accountability as a professional in the delivery of care and motivation of student nurses.

2. Identify organisational skills used in the clinical area.

3. Distinguish between the abilities of student nurses and identify their knowledge levels.

4. Recognise the value and importance of research in nursing care.

5. Know the importance of good communication at all levels and with all persons encountered.

6. Discuss the economic and political ideologies of the National Health Service.

Psychomotor
1. (a) Act in a professional manner at all times.
   (b) Acknowledge any limitations of competence and refuse in such cases to accept delegated functions without having first received instruction in regard to those functions.
   (c) Ensure that no action or omission that occurs on his/her part or within his/her sphere of influence is detrimental to the condition or safety of patients.

2. Appropriately delegate and organise individualised care.

3. Give instruction and supervision to student nurses.

4. Encourage all nurses to become research-minded and use the knowledge to promote optimum quality of care.

5. Display effective levels of communication at all times, appropriate to individuals encountered.

6. Utilise and teach the use of resources appropriately when organising the care of individuals.

Affective
1. Accept responsibility for his/her professional practice and development.

2. Accept her own role and responsibility for organisation of care and resources.

3. Appreciate the limitations of skills and knowledge level of student nurses.

4. Appreciate the value of research to enhance the quality of nursing care.

5. Accept that good effective communication is essential to harmonious relations.

6. Appreciate the value and show awareness of meticulous budget control in the National Health Service.

Index

Acknowledgements

Permission is acknowledged for use of material on the following pages:

p.13 Allan, P. and Jolley, M. (1981) *The Curriculum in Nursing Education*, p.29, London: Chapman & Hall.

p.17 Cybert, R.M. (1980) Problem-solving and education policy in Turna, D. and Reif, F. *Problem Solving and Education: Issues in Teaching and Research*, New Jersey: Erlbaum.

p.34 Allan, P. and Jolley, M. (1981) *The Curriculum in Nursing Education*, p.86, London: Chapman & Hall.

p.36 Boud, D., Keogh, R. and Walker, D. (1985) *Reflection: Turning Experience into Learning*, London: Kogan Paul.

p.40 Lawton, D. (1975) *Curriculum Studies and Educational Planning*, p.83, Sevenoaks: Hodder & Stoughton.

p.113 Quinn, F.M. (1988) *The Principles and Practice of Nurse Education*, 2nd edition, London: Chapman & Hall.